Practical Injury Prevention For Team Sports

How To Implement A World-Class System In Amateur Or Pro Sport Without Expensive Equipment

David O'Sullivan

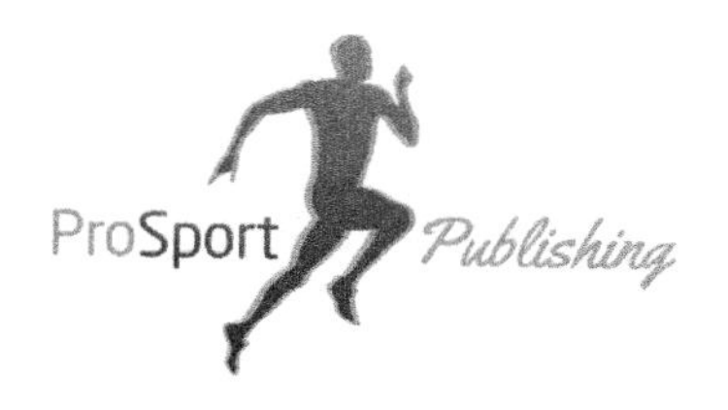

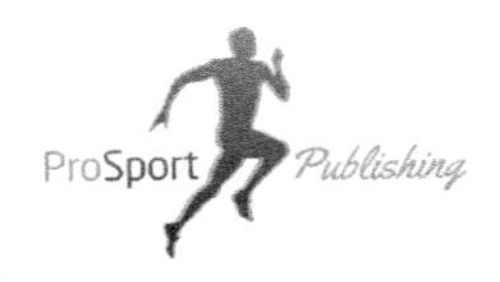

ISBN: 979 861302 110 9

A CIP record for this book is available from the British Library

Edited and typeset by Helen Jones

Facebook @TheProSportAcademy
Instagram @ProSportAcademy

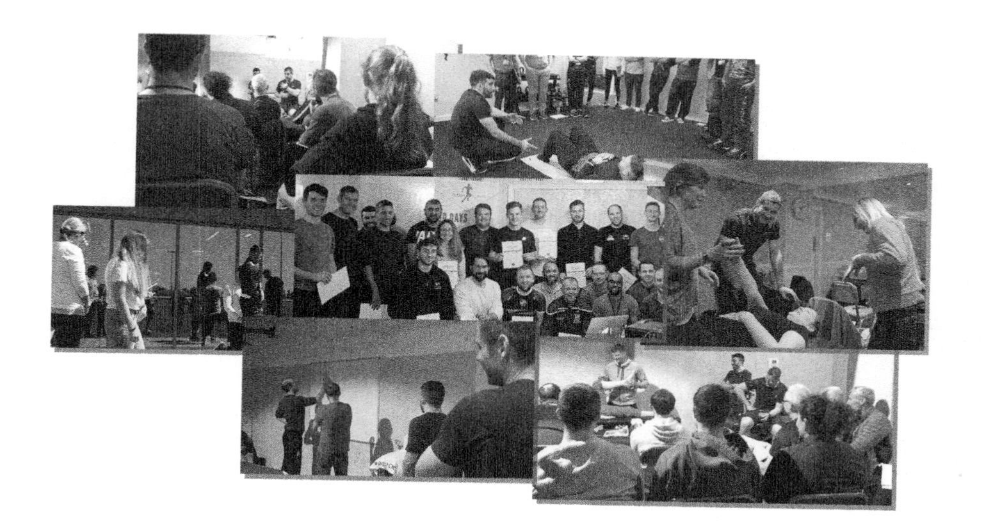

Dedication

For all the 'Go To' Therapist Mentorship students who took the leap and trusted me as a mentor. Thank you for keeping an open mind, moving outside your comfort zone, applying the content and continuing to evolve and improve the step-by-step system. I can honestly say as a result of your questions and as a result of watching how you are applying the content, I have improved as a clinician. Thank you.

Contents

You'll need this injury prevention pack as you work your way through the book

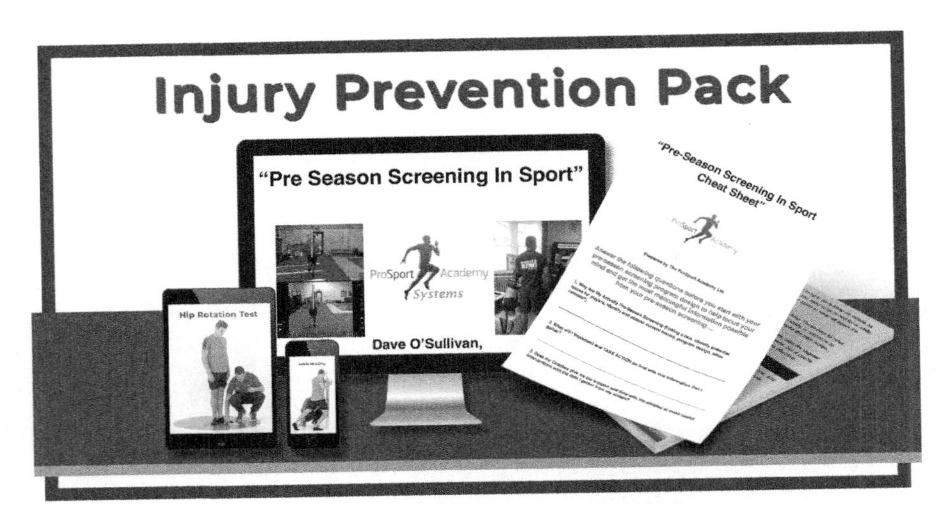

To unlock these free resources visit:
www.injurypreventionbook.com/resources

TESTIMONIALS

Bobby Sourbuts – England Rugby Physio
Working with the England team, our aim is to get the lads safely back on the pitch as quickly as we possibly can and keep them on there. Following Dave's system I was able to implement this straight away with the lads. I am much more confident now in saying 'yes, he'll be good to train today'.

Zeph Nicholas – West Indies Cricket Team Therapist
Dave's system has given me the confidence to treat anyone and not second-guess myself. I feel more confident that I can deliver the goods to put my patients in a much better place.

Philip Endl – Austria FC Under 21 Head Physio
Dave's system has given me a lot more confidence having a structure in place that I can rely on when treating. I can now deliver a complete treatment plan from start to end and have full confidence that my patients' pain will not return.

Almedin Muharemovic – Head Physio at NK Maribor FC Slovenia
Since implementing the system and getting great results my players started to trust me. I used to use a lot of machines but now I get better results with my hands and then I progress the player through the rehab using Dave's system and I trust in myself more and I am a lot more confident.

Shane Carney – Ulster Rugby Strength & Conditioning Coach
Investing the time to learn Dave's system has completely transformed my processes in delivery. He makes the complex so simple, and just as importantly scalable to all my athletes not just in one-to-one situations. This has allowed me to coordinate processes to ensure we have a robust injury prevention plan and also makes the stream from acute injury to return to performance seamless. It creates clear goals and markers which give athletes a vision of what they need to achieve to return quicker and become more robust than ever before. This gives both me and them the confidence to go for it on that journey but also the patience when things don't go as planned. In the never-ending and time-constrained world of sport the ability to have a system in place means that I can be deliberate and efficient with the time afforded, while also getting more consistent and better results than ever before.

Andy Barker – England FA Physio And Former Leeds Rhinos Head Physio
I was very fortunate to work with Dave in my first role following graduation at the Leeds Rhinos. I saw first-hand how he was able to implement strategies to get players back on the field faster than I ever thought possible and, not only that, get these players to not only survive, but thrive upon their return to action. Whilst the system he uses today has evolved greatly since we first worked together 10 years ago, I have seen how easy Dave's

content is to apply in the real world in both private practice and high level sport, getting quick results, but results that stick, and in the world of sport this is gold-dust.

Peter Connell – Huddersfield Giants First Team Sports Therapist
Dave's system is very easy to implement into everyday practice in professional sport. He has researched intensely and made the complex easy to understand and implement. The demands in professional sport are very high; using Dave's system I was able to get athletes back to training quicker than the 'standard protocols' and keep injuries down to a minimum using his injury prevention techniques.

Calum MacAskill – Ross County FC Head Physio
I've found Dave's system really beneficial; it has given me the tools and the confidence to put these protocols into practice with my players straight away and deliver great results.

David Roche – Physiotherapist For Irish Elite Olympic Athletes
Dave's system allows you to understand the real concise parts of rehab that you must go through to be confident in telling your patients when they can go back to the field of play, so there is no skipping stages which ultimately brings down injury rates.

Paul Cremin – London Irish RFC First Team Physio
I was fortunate that Dave gave me my first opportunity to work in professional sport. His mentoring and the implementation of his system gave me the clarity and confidence to work through even the most complex cases with a simple step-by-step approach. This provided some really quick results that players bought into really quickly. Dave's system really helped to accelerate my career in professional sport.

INTRODUCTION

At the end of 2012, I left my dream job at Munster Rugby Union and returned home to be with my then fiancée (now wife) Georgina and two-year-old daughter Ava May to head up the sports medicine team at Huddersfield Giants Rugby League Club.

I remember it well: the initial phone calls from the then club doctor sussing out my interest; then a Skype 'interview' with the head coach from my treatment room at the University of Limerick in Munster and then negotiating my contract with the CEO of the club while on pre-season training with Munster in France.

It was one of the hardest career decisions to make to leave my dream job so early but at the same time one of the easiest decisions as it meant I would return to be with my family in the UK.

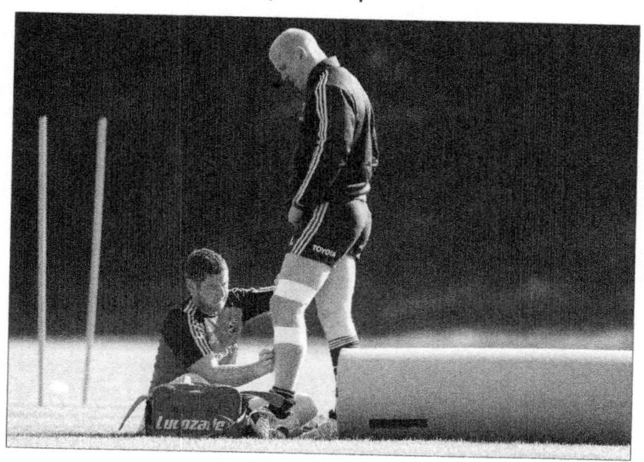

Working in my dream job at Munster Rugby, here with Paul O'Connell taking him through an MCL return to play session.

And so, with a heavy heart, I handed my notice in, packed the car up and got the ferry back to Huddersfield from Dublin on the 25th of October 2012.

The first of November was my official start date with the Giants and, on that cold morning, I went from the glam of the world class facilities of the Munster Rugby training ground at the University of Limerick to a private 'gym' (if you could call it that) and backroom of a shed that was to now be my physio room for the next 24 months at least. With that sub-standard and quite frankly inappropriate room, we had fold-up plinths, absolutely no budget or fancy equipment and just our hands and oil.

In addition to the gym and kitchen/dining room where we treated for a whole two years, I inherited 13 postseason surgeries and an injury rate in the double figures at the most important time of the year, the play-offs, which saw the team lose in the first round.

And the BIG thing about all this – I inherited this team from a super talented clinician that was doing all the right things on paper 'individual prehab sheets', 'wellness sheets', good hands-on treatment and an outstanding knowledge base. The clinician is still a leading clinician; I had worked with him previously and can still call him a friend to this day. The clinician had done all the right things and was in my opinion even ahead of the majority of therapists out there in the stuff that he had implemented, YET still had a surgery injury list that could fill a rugby league team sheet.

However, I had learned a thing or two from my four years with Leeds Rhinos, and my own mentor at the time Meirion Jones, and had also had the opportunity to work with a diverse range of strength and conditioning coaches at Munster Rugby, who all helped me improve as a clinician. I was finally ready to roll out MY injury prevention blueprint that had all but fallen into place after five years of being involved in pro sport, taking the best bits of the systems I'd worked with and refining them further as I continued to evolve, implement and, most importantly, learn from my own mistakes.

I was ready to take action and roll out a programme from scratch, with just a team of an assistant physiotherapist, a soft tissue therapist, a rehab strength and conditioning coach and me: our hands, a few bands, a few hurdles and our knowledge.

This blueprint was the result of hours and hours of reflection and trial and error while observing closely the mistakes and successes of not only my own work but the work of others.

And the results in the first 12 months?

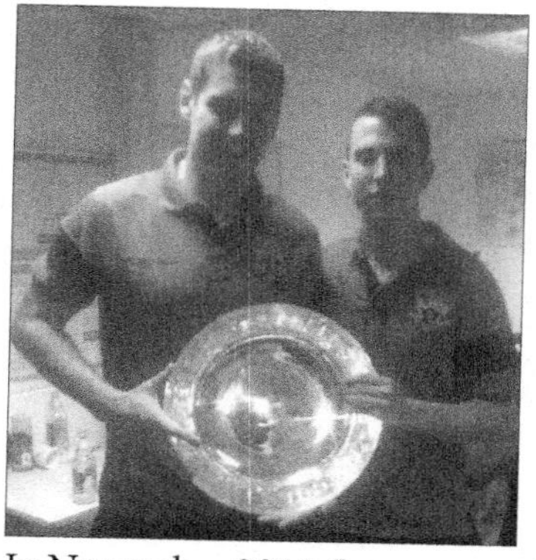

Here with assistant physiotherapist at the time, Darragh Sheehy. Huddersfield Giants won the League Leaders' Shield and their first silverware in over 80 years in 2013, our first season at the club.

In November 2013, I was returning for my second pre-season as Huddersfield Giants Head Physiotherapist with the lowest injury rates in Super League according to the University of Bolton Injury Surveillance Survey for the 2013 season (and subsequently the following two years); a league leader's shield that recognised us as the most consistent team in Super League in 2013 (the club's first silverware in over 80 years); and praise and recognition by players and staff both in private and in the public media for helping them achieve their own personal accolades.

I say this not to boast about myself (because this is not about me, this is about you) but rather to show you that with just a slight tweak in your way of thinking, some simple changes to things that are already happening at a club and developing a thought process that looks at the person rather than the injury, you can make changes very quickly.

At the start of 2018, I was asked by Warrington Wolves' then Head of Performance to get involved with Warrington Rugby League Club on a consultancy basis, working with their new head physio to mentor him and help him implement an injury prevention system.

Some simple changes in thought process, and an excellent working relationship and implementation between the medical department and the performance department at Warrington, resulted in them going from double figures in hamstring injuries the previous year to having one of the best injury rates in Super League in 2018 while reaching the Challenge Cup Final and Super League Grand Final in the same year.

I've also been 'lucky', if you can call it that, to be on the other end of this with another club recently where there was very little interaction between the medical, performance and coaching staff and the results were catastrophic during pre-season, which then filtered into the early results in the season. Some personnel changes and a healthy interaction and working relationship between medical, performance and coaching staff was able to overturn this (although it took some time) and the results again consistently go in the right direction.

This system is not rocket science. And, if you know anything about me by now, you know I like to keep things very simple and do the basics to an extraordinarily high level.

If you have your best players consistently on the field, then massive momentum can take place; even as underdogs with the Giants from 2013 to 2015, we never finished below third place in the regular season.

If you would like to discover the exact step-by-step common sense injury prevention system I used from 2013 to 2015 with the Huddersfield Giants, now help implement with other clubs I consult with and teach to my mentorship students all over the world, then grab a cup of coffee and keep reading...

But before we proceed, you should understand I have deliberately kept this book very conversational in its tone and manner. (This is similar to my other book, *The 'Go To' Physio.*) I have done this intentionally so as not to overwhelm you and to allow you to understand things easily so you can take action and implement what you learn in the real world.

I've no interest in sounding smart on paper if you cannot implement any of this in the real world. Everything I teach in my 'Go To' Therapist Mentorship is content that can be implemented the very next day and I want to keep this book the same so I have intentionally chosen to keep the language and grammar very simple.

Why an injury prevention system is critical in this day and age

Sports healthcare professionals have it tough… and it's getting tougher.

They have to undo the consequences of other people's actions and decisions: players, coaches and even strength and conditioning coaches.

They have to ensure that a group of athletes is not only able to recover after a game but is ready to train again in a day or so and ready to go 'to battle' again in sometimes less than five days.

They have to make decisions about if an athlete is ready to train with the team, what he/she can and cannot do and when to progress them to ensure that he/she is ready to go again in a few days' time.

Not only do they have to do this for one athlete but also sometimes for up to 50–60 athletes.

Sports healthcare professionals protect a club's or team's greatest assets yet need to push and push these assets without overstepping the mark and causing further injury or harm to an athlete.

A good sports healthcare professional that can interact efficiently with the performance department is indispensable to a club and will help the head coach by allowing him to choose his/her best team at the most important times of the year. A good sports healthcare clinician will help a strength and conditioning coach get the most out of an athlete and ultimately help them get the recognition they deserve.

And with the advances in sports science and coaches demanding that performance departments continue to push athletes even further than in previous seasons, it is no surprise that the majority of sports healthcare professionals are spending the majority of the time picking up the pieces.

And when you do pick up the pieces, you let the injuries or niggles settle, you may do your ultrasound, hands-on massage or cross frictions you were taught at university and you strengthen the muscles around the site of the injury and send the athlete back to train… only for the athlete sometimes to break down again a few days' or weeks' later. (And all of this is even happening with access to thousands and thousands of pounds/euros/dollars-worth of the latest technology for some therapists.) And the Head Coach, Performance team and even the players at times are passing judgement on you as a therapist.

Professional sport is challenging and, in the high performance environment, there is nowhere to hide: your results are on show for the world to see. This is why you need a robust system in place that takes into account modern pain and movement science that has to then be integrated with the performance department, to ensure the athlete is resilient when returning to their real world environment.

Although you may have worked hard studying to become a healthcare professional, worked endless hours studying and putting yourself out there on your path of trying to become recognised as one of the top therapists in the country by your peers, staff and athletes, you were never really told how to run a super-efficient, super successful injury prevention programme in the 'real' world of working in sport, be it amateur or professional.

I can help you to solve this problem and take away years of trying to figure this stuff out on your own. This book is written for you, to help you devise a successful, efficient injury prevention system that allows you to enjoy working with athletes and help them build resilience rather than simply papering over cracks and sending them back with no real clue if the athlete will 'break down' again.

With the confidence that not only have you addressed the 'true cause' of the athlete's injury but you also have a system in place to ensure that when the athlete returns to the team training environment, you have systems in place that will allow them to continue to build resilience.

And with that comes enjoyment going to work every day, knowing you are making a real difference to the team or athlete's chance of success and you receive gratitude and appreciation so that even if you or the athlete left the club, your value would be so well regarded that they would ring you up in a heartbeat if they ever were struggling with an injury or even if one of their new teammates were struggling to get right.

This system can easily be modified, even if you are a solo practitioner working in amateur sport or with individual athletes. This book will help you implement a system so that when the time comes for you and you receive your big chance of working in pro sport, you will be ready to take it and have a genuine understanding of how to implement an injury prevention system that will add massive value to the club or athletes you work with.

Do you really have an injury prevention system in place?

Most sports healthcare professionals will tell you they have an injury prevention system in place…

A pre-season screening that ends with a lot of paper in a drawer never to be seen again, or a few sets of rotator cuff or nordics thrown into a prehab programme. Or some may even consider doing some wellness and objective markers pre-training as an injury prevention system.

But to answer this question, we need to understand what a system truly is…

'A set of things working together as parts of a mechanism or an interconnecting network; a complex whole.' Google Dictionary, 2019

Or: ***A system is a group of interacting or interrelated entities that form a unified whole.' Wikipedia, 2019***

An injury prevention system needs to incorporate all the parts – from the medical, to the performance to the coaching department – in order to achieve the desired outcome: fit and resilient athletes that can perform to their athletic capabilities and be successful as a team or individuals.

I focus on 12 key components in my own injury prevention system which I'll outline in the first chapter. If you focus your attention on these 12 key components, then the results can be game-changing and will allow you to work smarter and not harder on a day-to-day basis.

CHAPTER 1

The 12 components of the pro sport academy injury prevention system

The reality is an injury prevention system is an ART rather than a science. There are so many things that have to fall into place for an effective injury prevention system so putting all your eggs in one basket will ultimately leave your system vulnerable.

With that said, I have identified 12 key components (or micro systems) that NEED to run well in order to have an effective injury prevention 'machine' or system that spits out strong, durable, resilient athletes.

There are always three micro systems that are overlooked that can cause many problems for sports healthcare clinicians moving forwards as the season unfolds.

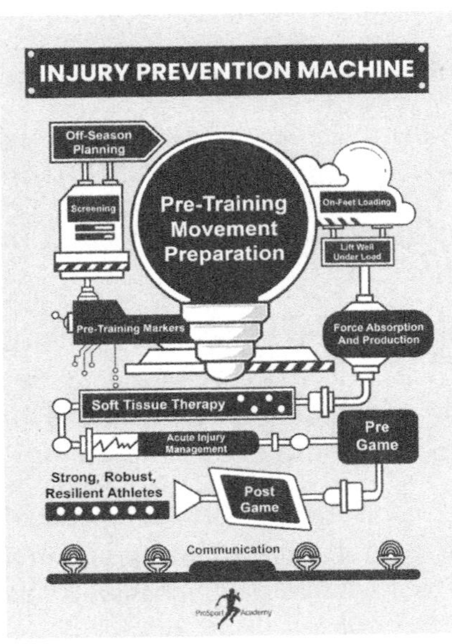

Before I dive into describing these problems, I want to outline what all of the 12 micro systems are that a leading sports healthcare professional needs to have in place, if they are to THRIVE in this new era of working in pro and amateur sport.

You see, the old ways of 'putting a bit of ultrasound', or using a little cross-friction or eccentrics just aren't cutting it anymore. The likes of Youtube, Google, Facebook and Twitter mean that there is so much information out there these days that players and coaches can stray and question your methods and techniques.

There is a massive OPPORTUNITY for up-and-coming sports physios and new age sports healthcare professionals like you and me to take a step back, acknowledge that our predecessors were doing the best they could and were applying their knowledge of the evidence in the sporting setting but appreciate that times have changed, training methods have changed and the demands placed upon us as healthcare clinicians and athletes have also changed.

The research and evidence is evolving and we are beginning to understand more about the motor adaptations to pain, how the body responds to stress and further insights into what muscles' true functions are, among many other great insights in the last decade.

Therefore we need a NEW WAY OF DOING THINGS, that will help us keep control of our squad and that will never have players or athletes doubting our methods: the results and benefits of our methods will be right there in front of them and for all the world to see.

Well, I'm going to show you how the new age sports healthcare professional takes action right now.

The 12 micro systems of The ProSport Academy Injury Prevention Machine takes into account the advances in the latest research, the advances in our understanding of the interaction between the various systems of the body and, most importantly, how all of this fits into the realities of working in sport, day in, day out.

Since I came out of working in full-time professional sport in October 2015, I have been helping therapists all over the world in both private practice and professional sport implement the NEW AGE Sports Healthcare Professional way of doing things.

And since working with leading physiotherapists, physical therapists, neuromuscular therapists, sports massage therapists, chiropractors and osteopaths in both amateur and professional sport, we have been able to really refine the injury prevention blueprint down to these 12 key components.

The Injury Prevention 'Machine' is all about working smarter rather than harder. It is about using the data and information we gather on a daily basis and allowing it to shape our actions. Individually some of the systems may look unrelated yet they all come together to help promote resilient athletes.

With that said, let's take a look at the 12 components:

1. The off-season planning micro system

This is where you identify your staff's strengths and weaknesses and ensure that every staff member is crystal clear on their role within the overall Injury Prevention programme. If your staff don't know their roles, or the consequences of them not doing the appropriate tasks each day, then you cannot identify where in the machine the problem lies that is ultimately spitting out an injured athlete. If you and your staff do not have clarity on your roles, then effective action is rarely taken. Gaining clarity has to be the first step.

2. The screening micro system

This is where you identify valuable pieces of information at key stages throughout the season that will give you meaningful data that is going to help you throughout the year with some key decisions. This will entail different screens at different times of year but the information gained will be indispensable to helping you going forwards and won't just be shoved into the filing cabinet, never to be seen again.

3. The pre-training markers micro system

This is where you will really zone in on potential issues on a day-to-day basis to ensure that no athlete 'breaks down' under your watch. This information will again be put to work in the accompanying systems and the days that follow, as well as helping with some key decisions and actions you and your team take.

4. The pre-training movement preparation micro system

This is where you will use all that meaningful information gained from the previous systems, in addition to information for further systems, to put together a movement preparation session that ensures each athlete's nervous system is primed for what lies ahead on this training day, avoiding protective tension, niggles or worse.

5. The on-feet loading micro system

This is where you will work closely with your strength and conditioning and performance staff to ensure you are working for the greater good of the team. This system will help you avoid protective tone, niggles and 'perceived threats' to the athlete's nervous system that will ultimately contribute towards injury and/or pain.

6. The 'move well under load' micro system

This is where you will ensure that all your hard work is not undone in a split second. This system will ensure that your athletes are not only moving away from pain but moving towards building resilient, robust bodies that can withstand the stresses that are placed upon them in the gym and on the field.

7. The force absorption and production micro system

This system ensures that you do not continue to pick up silly niggles when you send athletes back to training. This is arguably one of the most important pieces in the machine and helps you build strong, robust and resilient athletes. This system works closely with numerous other systems to be integral cogs in the machine.

8. The soft tissue therapy micro system

This system will ensure that when you or your team are performing hands-on treatment, it is helping and not hindering you. This will avoid you getting short-term reactions but long-term problems. This system will cooperate with various other systems to allow you to have a sniper rather than a bazooka approach identifying true causes and avoiding treating reactions with your soft tissue system in your club and your athletes becoming 'reliant' on hands-on treatment.

9. The acute injury management micro system

This is where you are going to ensure that little niggles and bangs do not turn into significant injuries and lost training days and time. You will also make certain that athletes do not pay the price for any injuries further down the line. While other clinicians are letting injuries 'settle', you will be taking time off the end stage rehab progressions by implementing a smart graded exposure programme from day 1 post injury which complements the healing process.

10. The pre-game micro system

This is where you get to enjoy the fruits of your week's work. You get to ensure that your athletes are prepped and ready to go and you can have a significant impact on your team's success on game day. This system allows a natural continuation of the working week and also ensures you don't fall at the final hurdle and pick up silly injuries on game day.

11. The post-game micro system

The post-game system allows you to go into the following day or week with less headaches, less stress and razor-sharp focus on what needs to be done in the coming weeks to ensure that you maintain a consistent and successful well-oiled Injury Prevention Machine.

12. The communication micro system

This system is one of, if not, the most overlooked system in every injury prevention programme. This system will allow you to ensure that the other 11 micro systems are working in total harmony to spit out a fit, healthy, strong, robust and resilient team that allows your coach to constantly pick their best players and your strength and conditioning coach to work with healthy athletes while you spend your time working with players that need your time and attention to ensure the overall success of the team. The coaching staff as a whole get to work smarter, not harder.

Why Do We Systematise?

They are several reasons why you'd want to systemise your injury prevention programme, but everyone misses the ultimate reason which I'll outline along with the other main reasons below.

1. Control the chaos

Working in sport brings its own challenges that university textbooks can't prepare you for. The reality is that once day 1 of pre-season starts, it is full-on until the last day of the season. Therefore having these systems in place allows for clarity and purpose with everything you do. It allows you to see the trees from the forest once the pressures of working in sport kick in. It also allows you to identify areas of the machine that need attention and your precious time is best spent on focusing or improving throughout the season.

2. Allows for accountability

This ties in especially with micro system 1. Every person in the team has a massive part to play in operating the Injury Prevention Machine. If an injury or issue does occur, having the systematised approach makes it extremely easy to quickly identify the key parts of the machine that need urgent attention and more importantly who is responsible for these parts performing well. This ultimately allows you to take action straight away before further injuries or issues occur.

3. Helps transition between staff members

Having systems allows new staff members to easily learn how the Injury Prevention Machine works and gives them clarity on what is expected of them to operate their parts of the machine. This allows for consistency in your Injury Prevention Machine, irrespective of staff members moving on. It also allows you to prioritise training new members in areas that will be important to them performing and contributing to the Injury Prevention Machine. It gives continuing professional development a new outlook, where you genuinely improve areas of a staff member's skill sets that will result in the greater good of the team and the individual.

4. Allows clarity for the end goal

The 12 individual micro systems allows for the utmost clarity in what needs to be done well in order to stand a chance of having a super-efficient and successful injury prevention system. The end goal is simple but the steps that need to be executed in order to get there can sometimes be vague. If every staff member knows their role and executes it, then you give yourself the best chance possible. Remember, a confused mind never moves forward.

5. A clear action plan to prevent injuries and do the basics extraordinarily

A system outlines clear action steps to achieve a goal. The system will allow you to take action now that everyone is clear on their roles. Most injury prevention programmes sound great on paper but are never put into action or followed through with consistency. The ProSport Academy's 'Go To' Therapist's 12 micro systems that ultimately are the Injury Prevention Machine allow you to do the basics extraordinarily and justify everything you are doing at any point in the season to get that ultimate result of less injuries and more durable, robust, resilient athletes that contribute to the team's overall success.

CHAPTER 2

The 'go-to' therapist sports healthcare professional

Before we get into the various parts of the machine, let's look at the driver of the machine: the 'Go To' Therapist. The 'Go To' Therapist doesn't accept dated explanations or old-fashioned 'it's just one of those things'. They are energised, enthused and hungry for knowledge and information; they question every injury. They make the most of opportunities to learn lessons from the failures in the present system and constantly question how they can do things better. Let's look at some of the characteristics of the 'Go To' Therapist:

The 'Go To' Therapist:

- ***Understands that pain is an output of the brain and does not simply mean damage to a tissue***

The 'Go To' Therapist understands that pain is a conscious experience and simply an output of the brain. The 'Go To' sports pro educates his/her patients on what pain is and what it is not.

The 'Go To' sports healthcare professional chooses their words carefully and does not simply use lazy language that ultimately may come back to haunt them later. They relate their explanations to the athlete in a meaningful way so the athlete can understand why their body may be organising itself in this way and why they are experiencing these unpleasant conscious sensations of pain, tightness etc.

The 'Go To' sports healthcare professional knows that there are many facets to the pain output experience and it is ultimately an interpretation from the body and brain from actual or 'perceived threats' to the system. They use this knowledge to their advantage when managing acute injuries to reassure athletes, which will ultimately help them cut time off the return to training times.

They also ask the simple question 'Why is this athlete's brain perceiving a threat at present?' taking into account the athlete's current home and working environment and previous days' and weeks' training loads and movements.

- ***Understands that stress precedes pain and can come in many forms***

The 'Go To' Therapist appreciates the role of stress or stressors on the body. They appreciate that stressors can be in numerous forms such as compensation strategies still in place due to previous injuries, emotional stressors placed on athletes as a result of team sporting environments, contract issues, family issues etc.

The 'Go To' Therapist understands that tissues such as the diaphragm and pelvic floor may react to such stressors with protective tone or muscle guarding and then influence the movement variability of the athlete. They appreciate that lifestyle stressors such as diet, sleep and other lifestyle choices can impact our ability to recover, our breathing rate and the ability to have variability between our heart rate, breathing rate and movement.

They appreciate how emotional and lifestyle stressors can alter the tone of the diaphragm and pelvic floor in anticipation to perceived threats or repeated bouts of trauma on the body such as contact training or sporting activities.

They appreciate the importance of the diaphragm and the pelvic floor's ability to lengthen and shorten in order to maintain movement variability, and how emotional and lifestyle stressors may have an influence on an athlete's movement options.

They appreciate that in the same way that nociceptors can become sensitised, so too can the chemoreceptors. This can affect the depth of our breathing which will affect the amplitude of diaphragm and pelvic floor movement and indirectly hence affect the musculoskeletal system such as thoracic mobility or pelvic mobility.

This knowledge will be essential when athletes present to the medical or performance department with consistently 'tight' hamstrings, calf muscles or low back muscles. The 'Go To' Therapist will avoid simply massaging or 'releasing' these but will have a thorough understanding of the underlying drivers specific to the individual.

- ***Understands that noxious stimulus can alter directions of force***

The 'Go To' Therapist understands that when there is a noxious stimulus to the system (think dead leg or bump to the leg in sport or prolonged conditioning drills that stress the nervous system to the max) the body goes about self-organising itself to be successful for that moment in time.

They understand that the athlete may not even have conscious awareness of the subtle differences in how their system has organised itself but the athlete will have altered their movement strategies as a result. They understand this could be significant when tracing back previous injuries and making sense of movement screens or how the athlete is moving here and now.

They will respect the injury history and the athlete's nervous system's attempts to keep the athletes successful in their sporting environment but understand that there may be a long-term consequence of such a strategy for the athlete on other tissues or joints that may become sensitised.

They will understand the value in restoring and reassuring the athlete's belief system in generating torque in particular directions and having intent to produce force in as many options as possible.

They will use this understanding to their advantage through various systems in the Injury Prevention Machine.

- ***Understands the generic reactions of the body to sympathetic dominance***

The 'Go To' sports healthcare professional appreciates that movement 'dysfunctions' or 'compensations' are simply strategies in reaction to pain or sympathetic dominance and not the true cause.

They understand that the athlete will attempt to succeed by using strategies such as excessively elevating the ribcage to overcome muscle slack in the mid-section. They understand this may then change the pelvic position and stimulate receptors around the skin, fascia and muscles of the hamstrings which may give the illusion of 'tight' hamstrings over time if this strategy is prolonged in the gym and during conditioning sessions.

They understand that athletes in sympathetic dominance will favour mouth breathing, have decreased amplitude of the diaphragm and pelvic floor during respiration which may or may not influence decreased movement variability, and decreased variance of movement through the full foot when moving both in the gym and when decelerating.

They understand that the way in which the athlete's body will self-organise will be entirely unique to that athlete/person and the true stressor is unique to them even though they may seem to move in similar ways to other athletes and present with similar symptoms.

The 'Go To' sports healthcare professional will strive to find the true stressors, no matter what system they are working on in the Injury Prevention Machine, and will no longer tolerate just treating the site of the issue and hoping for the best.

- ***Understands most technology readings are simply showing the reactions and not the true cause***

The 'Go To' Therapist understands that the scores from the objective markers and other modern technology are simply the outputs and results of how the person's nervous system has organised itself in the here and now. They understand that it is hard to assign cause and effect to one variable and that the whole body and person must be taken into account rather than just solely focusing on the musculoskeletal system.

The aim of the Injury Prevention Machine is to address the whole person and take everything into account so that we minimise the perceived 'negative' values showing up on our objective markers or modern injury prevention equipment.

It is beyond the scope of this book to go into these key principles in more detail, but for further reading and understanding of how to apply these principles, please refer to my other book *The 'Go To' Physio Book*. For evidence based literature on the above principles, please visit the reference list at the end of this book.

With that said, let's now move on and look at the vital cogs (or micro systems) in your Injury Prevention Machine.

For further reading on motor adaptations to pain or noxious stimulus, please see the reference section at the end of the book and also the latest research from Kylie Tucker, Paul Hodges and François Hug in particular.

CHAPTER 3

Off-season planning micro system

Upon reflection, one of the most useful things I did in October 2012 was to give clear goals and responsibility to my staff upon entering the Huddersfield Giants organisation. This should hold especially true in football with the number of healthcare professionals working in a sports medicine department increasing yearly.

The problem with increased numbers of staff is that we tend to lose accountability and we lose a lack of focus on what exactly our job is. Remember, a confused mind never moves forward.

In order for the first 'screw' to hold the machine in place, it is essential to spell out in no uncertain terms the three main jobs each staff member is predominantly responsible for.

This should also be the case even if there are just two staff members in your team or even yourself. Just do three things really well to begin with.

On a morning, or before training, there are usually four key areas that may require attention for the healthcare professional and these need to be addressed efficiently for a successful Injury Prevention Machine to work well.

1. **Acute Injuries/Niggles**
2. **Long Term Rehab Players**
3. **Soft Tissue Prescription Of Healthy Athletes (Massage)**
4. **Pre-Training Markers**

For example, with the Huddersfield Giants I was lucky to have a sports therapist, an assistant physiotherapist and a strength and conditioning/ sports therapist rehab conditioner working with me.

The roles were as follows every morning:

Head Physiotherapist:

1. Acute injuries/niggles on a daily basis first thing in the morning plus communicating these, and any training limitations for any player, to the head coach.
2. Lead movement prep sessions with squad based on information gained from pre-training markers micro system and after discussion with the performance department on the content for the day's field session.
3. Treat long-term rehab players.

Assistant Physiotherapist:

1. Treat acute injuries for younger squad members or players who are unlikely to be considered for this week's game.
2. Monitor online subjective wellness and objective markers in mornings (dedicated time blocked off in diary to do this daily pre-training) and communicate findings to head physio and performance department if required.
3. Physically speak to players face to face and provide a hands-on assessment of any players who fell below baseline markers and did not resolve with conservative treatment/restoration exercises.

Sports Therapist: Soft Tissue Lead:

1. Manage soft tissue diary of players and prescription of soft tissue treatments bespoke to the person.
2. Oversee team of masseurs as required and ensure soft tissue therapy micro system implementation.

Sports Therapist: Rehab Conditioner:

1. Hydration scores of squad.
2. Additional movement sessions with players identified as needing additional work such as additional deceleration work or hip work etc.

3 **Weights and conditioning with long-term injured players.**

This way of working means that from 7am to 9am in the morning, all players are catered for and realistic gains can be made every day.

Let's break this down further. As a head physiotherapist, I don't need to worry about wellness scores being done: I know there is a person responsible for this. If a player does not have these done, then I know exactly who I need to speak to in my staff if the head coach addresses me with this. The assistant physiotherapist oversees this and physically gets their hands on players who are below baseline.

We do not 'trust' the players to do the right thing because we know the reality of the situation which is that players can become distracted so easily in a team setting. So, even though we should be able to rely on them to get these done, we don't take the risk. We schedule time in the assistant physiotherapist's diary, because what gets scheduled gets done.

I can focus entirely in the mornings in ensuring that I get players who are required for the weekend to be right and available for selection. This gives me the best chance of helping any who may have picked up some form of protective tone to be ready for the weekend or the training session ahead and to prevent these issues from developing further.

The soft tissue therapist is also ensuring that the players are getting the correct stimulus to their tissues and not simply further sensitising peripheral tissues for the sake of it. The soft tissue therapist ensures that the players pre-training markers are done before treatment sessions and the stimulus is meaningful to that athlete in helping them get back to baseline or homeostasis. This is invaluable in stopping me having to deal with issues later in the day after training or after protective tone has got worse.

The rehab conditioner can then focus on addressing our concerns with players' movement potential in the form of a small group of players who may need additional attention or help with cueing. This may happen daily, biweekly or weekly depending on our concerns. The content will usually focus first and foremost on improving the ability to absorb force and in developing athleticism. This is notoriously the new signings who had not been in our movement system previously and are noticeably behind in terms of deceleration and absorbing force with efficiency compared to the main squad.

In two hours in the above scenario, the amount of 'quality' work that has been done for various squad members is paramount but, most importantly, the data we have picked up from our key screws are utilised at every opportunity possible so no data is wasted or done for the sake of it.

You will be surprised how your motivation will change and you will make sure things are done well when you have complete clarity on your role and are only responsible for one or two things rather than the work being spread across the department loosely.

Ultimately, this is a high performance environment and there are consequences for our actions or inactions. Once we know who's responsible for whatever is not being done efficiently, if things don't go right, we know exactly who is not playing their part, and can address this.

Now, while that may sound a little bit cruel, it's not set out like this to catch anybody out, but it's simply to ensure that if there is a screw loose within the machine, we can easily find the screw and tighten it up again.

The most overlooked job role in off-season planning

The most overlooked job role in the off-seasoning planning is the person responsible for pre-training markers from my observation of pro sports medicine teams. This screw is arguably the least technical but almost critical for any machine to run well. In my instance, this screw was tightened by my assistant physiotherapist. From 40-45 minutes prior to our movement prep or training session starting, they were solely responsible for the pre-training markers being completed by players and also getting their hands physically on any players whose pre-training markers were down within 10 per cent of their baselines.

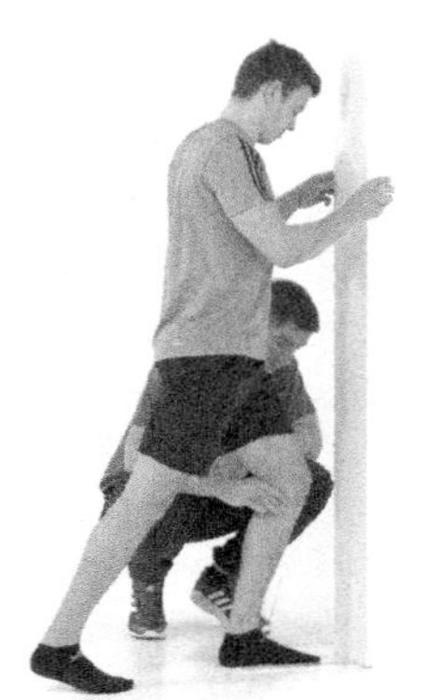

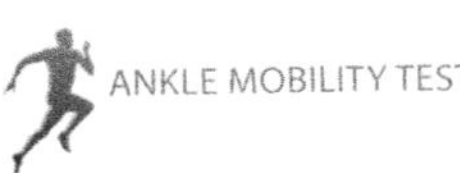

Taking an athlete through the ankle mobility pre-training test.

I will touch on this in the pre-training micro sections in a lot more detail. Both from my experience and observing many professional clubs, too many clubs are happy just to have the exercises printed out on the wall and then basically assume that the athlete is going to do the pre-training markers and then once their baseline is down that they're going to diligently go and do the exact exercises that are on the wall.

Well, unfortunately I can tell you from experience that may happen for two to three days but once the novelty wears off and the reality of the real world sets in, athletes get distracted. There is dressing room banter, there are coaches grabbing the athletes for a quick chat. There is always something going on in the morning before training starts. Therefore, do you realistically expect that athlete to do that on their own? In my experience, that just does not happen (for the majority of the squad anyway; there will always be the exception).

Having a dedicated member of staff, where they block their diary off to solely focus on this for 30-40 minutes before training is the only way to do this well from my experience.

Now, depending on the amount of restriction or reduction in the range of motion or symptoms, that athlete may actually physically get 5–10 minutes of manual intervention and then will be directed to some specific stuff based on what that therapist found, or if the athlete had an explanation for why they were down, then the assistant therapist would then direct them to one or two exercises under supervision.

This personal communication cannot be underestimated and is absolutely essential. The ability to get your hands on somebody and double check their scores and then find out WHY the pre-training markers are the way they are is also absolutely essential.

I've no doubt when I made this small change it had big rewards throughout the full year.

Soft tissue therapy pre-training

The soft tissue therapist's sole responsibility is the hands-on treatment of soft tissue; not only that, they ensure that every player gets what they need rather than what they want.

The 'Go To' healthcare professional understands that most tightness is simply receptors becoming sensitised and contributing to giving us some conscious awareness that these tissues are operating at a different threshold from how they usually would.

Receptors will be stimulated when lengthening, therefore further lengthening these tissues such as the hamstrings never quite made sense to me when someone had 'tight' hamstrings. Helping other tissues to restore their lengthening ability will usually give back movement options to the system and decrease the sensitivity of the original tissues, from my clinical observation.

One of the biggest changes I made when I went to Huddersfield Giants in late 2012 was to ban players from getting their lower backs and hamstrings rubbed because routinely players would come in, lie on their front, say that their hamstrings and lower backs were 'tight' and they'd get them massaged. There was no asking the question: Why are these tissues contributing to this conscious unpleasant experience of 'tightness'?

Why are the receptors and the tissues around the hamstrings and lower back giving this signal to the higher centres of the brain that is then interpreted as this conscious experience?

Until we start to ask why and make sense of the person's story in front of us, then we have no business putting our hands on players. Simply treating tissues that are 'tight' in isolation without any clinical reasoning makes athletes vulnerable to craving these short-term reflexive changes and becoming reliant on hands-on treatment and less independent.

Now, this may seem a bit extreme but if you want a world-class injury prevention system then make sure the screws are tight because it may be a long bumpy season ahead…

The information that we get from pre-season screening, which I will talk about in the next section is put to good use by the soft tissue department. My own soft tissue therapist had some clear instructions and they knew exactly what was happening with their mini department based on the data they were getting from our pre-season screening or pre-training markers and our in-season screening. No pre-season screening or daily markers data was ever put inside a filing cabinet and left to sit there. If we tracked something, then we made sure we used that data to our advantage and considered it in the general overall picture.

The rehabilitation specialist was working from information we picked up in pre-season and in-season screens but also from observing players in the gym and in the movement prep sessions. There were clinically reasoned explanations for everything we'd done with a player before training.

Another reason why I felt we got massive gains and results from our Injury Prevention Machine was the ability of every team member to have clear actions, to have clear consequences for their actions and also to know exactly what their job role was. There were no cookbook approaches used of just doing something for the sake of it.

It wasn't a case of 'Whoa… well, I thought *you* were going to do it today'. We, as a department, took responsibility for the movement prep sessions, which in previous years the strength and conditioning coach may sometimes have taken. But as soon as I got there, I took responsibility for it and I put structures and strategies in place which I will share with you in this book.

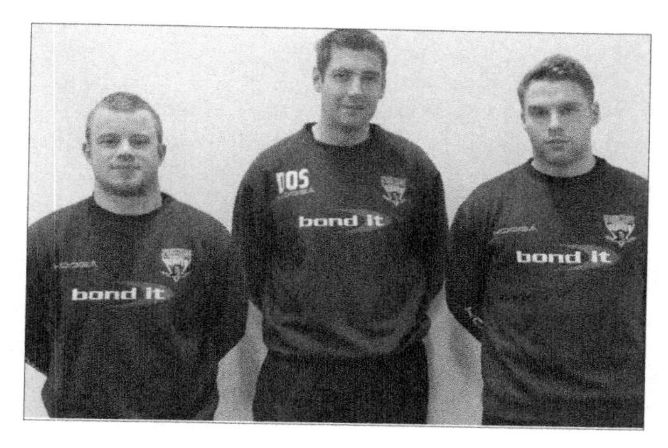

Here with my medical team at the start of my final season with the Huddersfield Giants in 2015. Aly McFarland on the left who was assistant physiotherapist at the time and Ollie Waite, who was the soft tissue specialist and rehab physiotherapist. Our injury prevention system was very successful again in 2015 due to the well-oiled interaction between the three of us and the performance team. Both therapists have gone on to have very successful careers as they climbed the promotion ladder.

Summary of key points

Organising my own and my team's job roles and responsibilities was one of the best decisions I made; it gave everyone a clear focus where everybody knew where they stood. So organising your staff and having clear intent on their daily tasks is essential. For the single practitioner working in amateur sport, organising your hour or two before training to some modified form of the above may be invaluable in chipping away at tightening up that screw in your own Injury Prevention Machine.

CHAPTER 4

Screening micro system

Screening and especially pre-season screening is usually perceived as some magical time of year where a lot of physiotherapists get really excited. It is indeed always an area where we always get a very big response whenever we do our pre-season screening webinars at **thegotophysio.com**.

Now, one thing that I would say is that this can either be a very valuable time of year or can be a massive tripwire for clinicians. They may have spent upwards of seven plus hours a day for two or three days gathering all this data and the reality is, by the end of the second or third day, even though it was the first week of pre-season, they're absolutely exhausted. They've lost motivation. They end up going through the motions and usually the data just gets put into the cabinet.

Another point to note is movement is task-specific and relies heavily on intent. We need to be careful of making assumptions based on the results of the movement screen whatever these may look like or of being too quick to try to 'correct dysfunctional movement', whatever 'dysfunctional' movement is.

The environment, the interpretation of information received from the eyes, the task or outcome that the athlete is focusing on will all have implications on how the body chooses to self-organise to complete this specific task or movement. Therefore this movement strategy may look completely different in different sporting situations, with different consequences for the brain.

You need to be careful to appreciate this when interpreting your results, in my opinion. With that said, screening can give us valuable information when used smartly.

The screening 'screw' has five corners:

1 Pre-season

2 In-season

3 Movement prep

4 In the gym

5 On the field

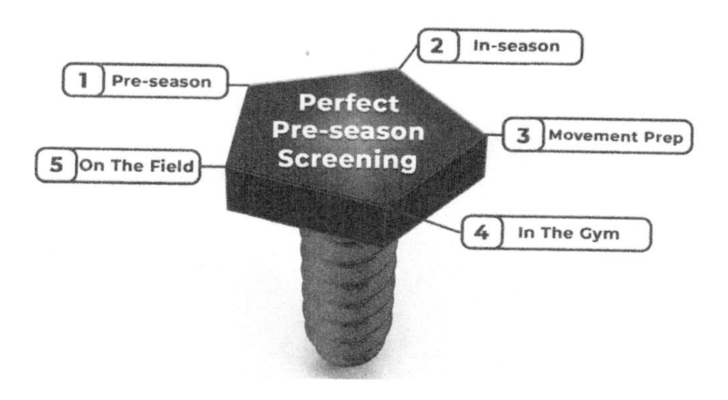

Pre-season screening

If you plan pre-season screening right, you can spend as little as two hours physically screening 30 athletes and get enormous amounts of information that can be used right through the season.

I've got to that point by having to figure out some key lessons that I'm about to share with you now so you can avoid making the mistake of spending hours upon hours of screening, that basically ends up squashed into a filing cabinet.

The biggest lesson that I want to share is this…

When you design your pre-season screening, most therapists I know perform an analysis for their chosen sport. The REALITY is that pre-season training is a time when your team will do almost anything but their sport for long periods.

If you work in Rugby Union, Rugby League and to some extent football, pre-season is a unique time of year; ultimately the pre-season screen should screen for suitability of a player to perform their duties over the coming weeks rather than how they perform their sport.

For instance, during this time of year athletes will commonly perform longer duration runs, higher intensity loads in the gym, different movements such as MMA or wrestling classes or even army camps. Your screen ultimately needs to show suitability for these movements and activities that the athlete is about to undertake during the next block, not movements specific to their sport that they will be performing during in-season.

In a nutshell, whether right or wrong, the reality is the main aim of the medical department during pre-season should be to 'survive' and minimise the number of soft tissue injuries accrued and allow the players to participate in as much of the pre-season training as possible. When we appreciate the impact previous injuries can have on future injuries and the importance of athletes having some form of chronic load under their belts, 'surviving' pre-season can have a massive impact on reducing injuries accrued during in-season, in my opinion.

If you get this screening right, then you will be able to identify in some way those athletes that need some immediate attention for the demand that their body is about to go through in the pre-season period.

Your sporting analysis will usually take place before your in-season screen, but for now focus on what your athlete will go through over the next six to eight weeks.

Choosing your screening movements

When we choose a particular series of tests, they should serve a very useful purpose and give us as much data as possible that can be used across numerous micro systems in order to make that time spent screening meaningful.

I personally want the data to help me with the following throughout the season:

1. **Pre-training markers baseline scores**
2. **Objective range of motion markers that can be used when an athlete has an acute injury to help me get them back to this, post-injury**
3. **Data that will help me make informed decisions about the content of my movement prep sessions**
4. **Data that will help me have meaningful conversations with the strength and conditioning team about a player's suitability to perform key lifts under heavy loads**
5. **Data that will identify any player with pain performing any of the movements I deem important for that athlete to be successful.**

So, from the above, you will choose three to four movements that will straight away double up as pre-training markers. You will also choose three to four more movements that you may use as objective range of motion tests if injuries do occur pre-season or in-season so you have some idea what the range of motion or result of such tests were before the athlete underwent pre-season. Then choose some body weight movements (for example) of variations of key lifts the athletes will perform during pre-season in the gym.

That leaves room for a few more tests that may help with how athletes are self-organising with regards absorbing force to help identify the level we start at with our movement prep sessions.

Here are some of the questions I use that may help you identify and focus your attention on which movements should be included in your screen:

1. **Where are the key stressors going to come from during the next six weeks (or whatever the duration of pre-season screening is) for this player?**
2. **What are the key movements in the gym that the athlete will be doing in pre-season?**

3 **What are the key movements the athlete will be doing in the next six weeks that will involve some form of contact training during wrestling, boxing, strongman etc?**

4 **What are the key movements in the next six weeks that the athlete will be doing for their conditioning (short and sharp sprints with up/downs or long continuous running or conditioning games?**

5 **Have ALL my athletes been exposed to these movements from answers two to four previously?***

Movements such as the 'knee to wall lunge test' can be extremely useful in giving some form of baseline score with an athlete of what they are able to achieve before they start training. As the season progresses, the player may pick up an ankle injury, for instance, but we can quickly take that data and go, 'OK. Your knee to wall is six now after the injury. Your knee to wall is only seven on your non-injured side, but actually when I checked your data from pre-season screening, you actually had 9cm of knee to wall on this side.' So we have some form of baseline we can refer to throughout the year; after an injury we can strive to restore the once available range of motion for the athlete.

Some form of hip rotation test, and some form of generic shoulder range of movement tests, can also be quite useful as they can also double up as objective markers when we are making decisions on when a player is returning to play or progressing to the next section of the rehabilitation.

*For a full list of the questions I ask myself related to my own screens and other movements I like to use, please visit **http://www.injurypreventionbook.com/resources**

A good rule of thumb for deciding on your tests is this: If you can't teach a test to a student or even to somebody involved with the team, whether it's a coach, the kit man or whoever, and they can't perform that test for you after you explain it to them, then, I may argue, is it a reliable test?

Pre Season Screening Rationale		
Test	Why	Cross Reference
Knee To Wall	Baselines, ↓ DF ↑Force via hip,knee and Lx spine. <10cm ↑ Risk of Injury.	Squat , SL Squat (Rule out =>Glute Med.), Depth Jump (=>Glute Med.) Toe Touch),
Hip Extension Test	↓ Poor Treble Extn, Ability of Quads to Lengthen; Hamstring, Groin, Lx Spine	Squat (Pelvic Tilt), Bridge Core (Inhibition), SL Squat (Tilt), OH Reach (Tilt), Toe Touch (tilt).
Body Weight Squat	Universal Ready Position, Ability to load safely	OH Reach Test (Rule out Low Limb Pelvic compensations), Hip Extension (Rule out Prox. Restricion =>Distal Quads Issue). SL Squat (L Vs R issue), Ankle Mobility (Rule out ankle issue), Depth Jump (=>NMSK if Squat OK).
Single Leg Squat	Landing/Deceleration Ability, Frontal Pelvic Stability, Lower Limb Alignment	Ankle Mobility (Rule out ankle =>Glute Med) Hip Extension Test (Inhibition Glute Max), BW Squat (NMSK Issue), 1 Legged Bridge (Check Glute Med in this, if ok in bridge=>? Adductors).
OH Wall Reach	Ability Overhead Lifting w/out compensation=>Lats, Pec Minor or Quads	Squat (Rules out Quads), Retest in Standing =>Rules out Lats, Indicated Pec Minor
Aspleys Scratch Test	Ability to display Flex/Ext Rotn and Extn/Int Rotn. Assess Shoulder Extension for Sprinting	OH Reach Test Clears Pec Minor/Sternal Fibres Pec Major And Lats for Flex/Ext Rotn
1 Legged Bridge	Ability of Glute Medius and Contralateral Obliques Co Contract	Hip Extension Test (Inhibition Glute Max), SL Squat (Indicates Obliques if SL Squat OK), Toe Touch OK =>? Glute Medius Issue as Core is firing
Toe Touch	Ability Post. Wght Shift,Lumbopelvic Rhythm, Hip Mob, Lx Sp. Force distribution	Ankle Mobilty (Mainly PF but ankle centration), Hip Extension Test (Rule quad length, tilt), BW Squat (hip mob), Bridge Core (Cocontraction Obliques n Glutes)
Depth Jump	ACL Indicator of ↑Risk, Deceleration Issues (tendons), Adductor Overload on conc.	Ankle Mob (Rule out=>?Glute Med), BW Squat (Pelvic or hip Issue rule out), SL Squat (Rule out Glute Med=>? Adductor,
Adductor Squeeze	Adductor Baselines for Season Ahead, Indicate Lumbopelvic Issues	↓, Use BW Squat Adductor Magnus Restrictions, Depth Jump for Overload Issues, Hip Extension Test for Hip Decentration Issues
Rotator Cuff Testing	Baselines for Season, Looking anything less than 20kg, Potential At risk Players SLAPs	OH Reach Test to check for Shoulder Joint Decentration
Postural Restoration Classification	Improve Ability of Left AF IR, ↓ Hip Labral Tears, Hernias, Lumbopelvic Issues	Hip Extension Test (Rule out Quads Issues with Modified Extension Drop Test).

"MOVE WELL IN THE GYM => MOVE WELL ON THE PITCH"

Here is an example of a document I put together for the 2013 pre-season along with the rationale for each test. With each of the tests we wanted to ideally be able to cross-reference these tests with the others to help us rule in or rule out certain parts of the body as potential drivers for a problem as it relates to the athlete's personal story and injury history.

What you want to do when choosing your pre-season screening is to pick easy tests that can be replicated any place, any time. That's going to be pretty important and useful for you when you decide on your pre-training markers.

The number of tests ultimately is going to be dictated by the amount of information you need in order to check the suitability of your players to do pre-season screening. For instance, I know in Rugby Union and Rugby League that the players are going to be placed under massive amounts of stress both physically and mentally over the next six to eight weeks. I know the positions that they have to get into in order to be successful and my screens need to take these into consideration.

However, before I decide on my exercises to include in my own screen, I need to know some other vital information.

I need to know the type of conditioning that the athletes are going to undertake. For example, is the type of running the conditioning team will be putting the athletes through predominantly aerobic focused or anaerobic focused? What are the postures the athletes will be required to sustain for prolonged periods under both physical and mental fatigue?

I need to understand the type of drills that the athlete will do in the wrestle session or the contact sessions. I need to be confident the athlete can again physically get into these positions or, looking at it another way, can their tissues lengthen and shorten without protective tone, in order to be successful in these positions? Is there a movement that will stress these tissues that may give us clues that there might be a problem?

I also need to know the key lifts that the strength and conditioning coach plans to do with the athletes during pre-season. Is an athlete able to get into a good deadlift or Olympic lift start position? If the athlete is unable to do this due to protective tone or some other reason, then do they really have any business doing this in the gym at this moment in time under near maximal loads? Would they be better served short-term using a plate/block under the bar on each side initially to allow them to start in a better position, or is there a physical intervention my team can help with to allow the athlete to be successful in the gym? I hope you can now see how I am using this information to help the strength and conditioning staff be successful but also to stop issues before the athlete even begins training.

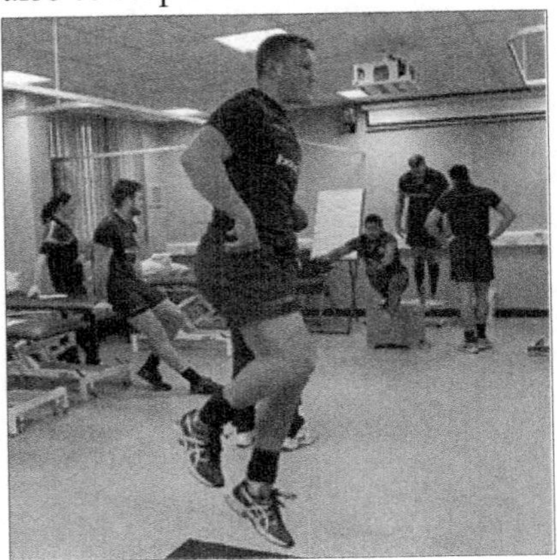

Players undertake movements that they will be required to do during the pre-season period.

Really, until I know all the information above, I believe I have no real business designing a pre-season movement screen. If I design a pre-season movement screen that's just solely focused on my needs, then ultimately I'm not checking the suitability of my athletes to go in and safely conduct this six to eight week period of training under extraordinary loads both mentally and physically.

Executing the screen

You want to set up your pre-season screening so that it literally can be replicated within two hours easily, multiple times throughout the season. If your pre-season screening takes a whole day or more to implement, the chances are you will not be able to repeat this screen or have availability (or time) to re-screen and re-evaluate your athletes through the season. If you asked a coach not to train on a particular day in-season because you want to re-screen your whole team, how do you think that would go down? This is why it's essential that it's quick and easy to replicate.

A successful Injury Prevention Machine is going to require you to screen your athletes at least twice throughout the year; therefore you need to make this as easy and stress-free for you as possible.

You can achieve this by getting a group of 10-12 students (sports science, physiotherapy etc.) to help you by supervising the individual screens or as a last resort even have the squad partner to supervise if working in amateur sport.

The point is this: for an effective screen, you should be able to grab family members, kit men, anyone you have available and have them help you screen all squad members easily.

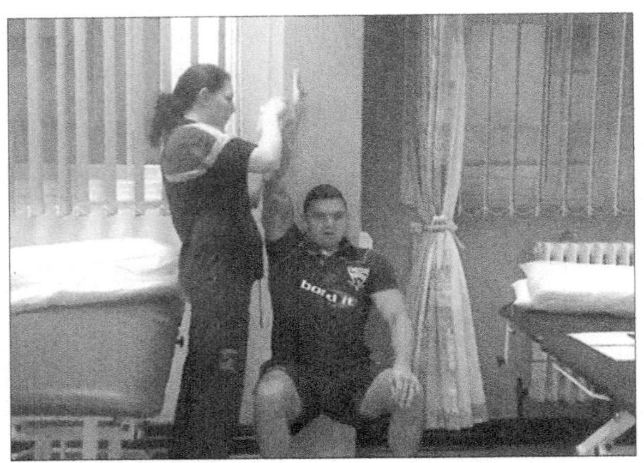

Here is a student performing a very simple screen to assess for any limitations in shoulder flexion.

If you are looking at body weight movements such as single leg squats for depth or body weight squats or deadlift start positions, just having an iPad or smartphone is of enormous benefit. A student or friend under clear instructions can simply record from the angle you instruct and you or your team can simply fly through the videos after the screen. Remember, you are looking for elephants not mice with all these screens so even going through the whole squads single leg squats for instance should take one to two minutes max per player.

Understanding the limitations of most injury prevention screens out there to accurately predict injury should not deter us from using pre-season screens as we can use this data for multiple reasons and not worry about every little piece of a movement but just have a bird's-eye view of each player and if something flags up, then better spend our time working with a player who needs it.

We can score the athlete using a number system of 1-3 with some predefined values like other screens use (such as functional movement screen) but we will use these scores simply as a means of communication to help us identify quickly where the player is at. I like to personally colour-code each score red, orange or green and this will help me get an easy visual on where my squad is at as a whole and it will become pretty clear what I need to focus on with my pre-training preparation movements and soft tissue treatment prescription.

We don't worry too much about the 1, 2 or 3 scores and trying to diagnose based on these scores. These simply allow us to get a bird's-eye view rather than making assumptions based on these scores.

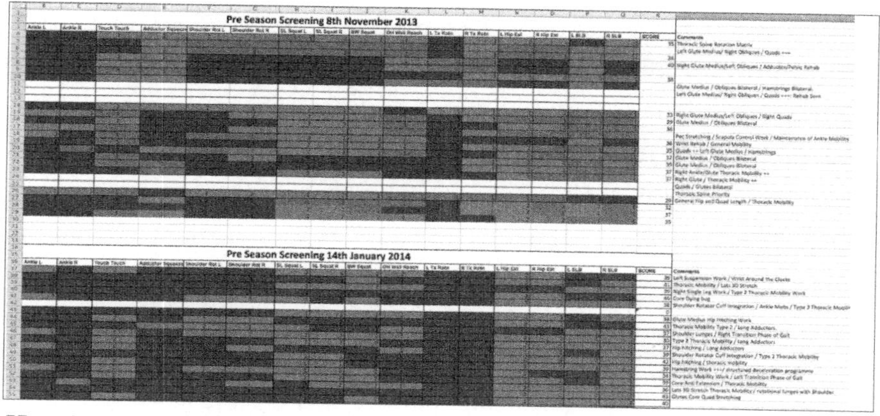

Pre Season Screening 8th November 2013

Ankle L	Ankle R	Touch Touch	Adductor Squeeze	Shoulder Rot L	Shoulder Rot R	SL Squat L	SL Squat R	BW Squat	OH Wall Reach	L Tx Rotn	R Tx Rotn	L Hip Ext	R Hip Ext	L SLB	R SLB	SCORE	Comments

Pre Season Screening 14th January 2014

Ankle L	Ankle R	Touch Touch	Adductor Squeeze	Shoulder Rot L	Shoulder Rot R	SL Squat L	SL Squat R	BW Squat	OH Wall Reach	L Tx Rotn	R Tx Rotn	L Hip Ext	R Hip Ext	L SLB	R SLB	SCORE	Comments

Here is an example of what my spreadsheets would look like at the start of pre-season and just before in-season. The colour coding helps focus on areas that may need attention during movement prep sessions and when receiving soft tissue treatment on a weekly basis.

When we analyse the scores we need to be careful not to make assumptions based on what's causing this score. We will utilise the whole screen combined with the athlete's previous injury history to make more of an informed decision rather than putting it down to a 'weak glute medius' for example. (Why is that glute medius displaying a decreased motor output? would be a better question to ask yourself.) We can still get consistent information about where the athlete was before they start their training, our pre-season training and where they are at now on a daily basis.

Your 4-key daily pre-training markers (which we'll cover in another section) should ultimately form a key section of the pre-season screening. You may then add in some other forms of test, for instance, a body weight version of the key lifts that they are going to do under load in the gym, as well as some form of general mobility test that tests the ability of the athlete's upper body to shorten and lengthen while their lower body may have faced a different direction. Some form of test that stresses the variance of movement of the athlete is always a good option, in my opinion.

From here then, we are testing the ability of the system to take up muscle slack, to self-organise and ultimately to ask the question: Does this athlete have the movement capabilities to execute these exercises safely both in bodyweight as in games and under load as in the gym situation?

Does this athlete have the ability to put forces in as many specific directions as possible and, ultimately, is this athlete robust?

From my experience, if the athlete moves well in the gym, then they will move well on the field.

Pain with screening

If your athlete indicates pain in any test, then this would be a big red flag and this will be an athlete we definitely want to focus some individual attention on. Pain means there is an interpretation of a 'perceived threat' and there is a perceived problem already present in this patient's nervous system that they will be probably be working around and adapting to at present. We understand the interaction between pain and movement and will want to inspect this 'perceived threat' further.

Do not simply accept this pain and brush it aside. Invest why there is a perceived threat and take action straight way.

In-season screening

The beauty of using this approach and being able to screen a team in less than two hours is that the in-season or end of pre-season re-screen can be executed even quicker.

For example, the athletes will be able to self-administer four of your tests in the form of the pre-training markers. The remaining tests will then be focused on what lies ahead and follow the same format as the pre-season screening:

- **What key lifts will the athlete be performing in the gym?**
- **What key movements or what directions of stress will the athlete be exposed to in training and in games?**

- **What contact drills or contact movements in games will the athlete be exposed to during the next block?**

While the majority of the screen may stay the same, a couple of tests may change depending on the answers to the questions above.

The in-season screen also serves an important purpose in helping you refocus and redefine your movement prep programme design while also updating modifications that athletes have been using in the gym.

Other opportunities to screen

This should go without saying but you will always be observing your athletes and asking why. Why is the athlete using this current movement strategy and how does it relate to their own story? The ability to 'see' an athlete moving with a high threshold, rigid strategy in movement prep sessions, in the gym or on the field is essential also and action needs to be taken to investigate further.

Cross-referencing screens

The doctor may carry out their own screens (for the heart, for example). The strength and conditioning coach may perform their own screens or testing and it is important to cross-reference the results so you have an overall picture of your athletes. Your screen should complement and build on the information and data gained from other departments. The results in the strength and conditioning screen should make sense with what you see based on your own screen if you appreciate how the body will self-organise to achieve tasks.

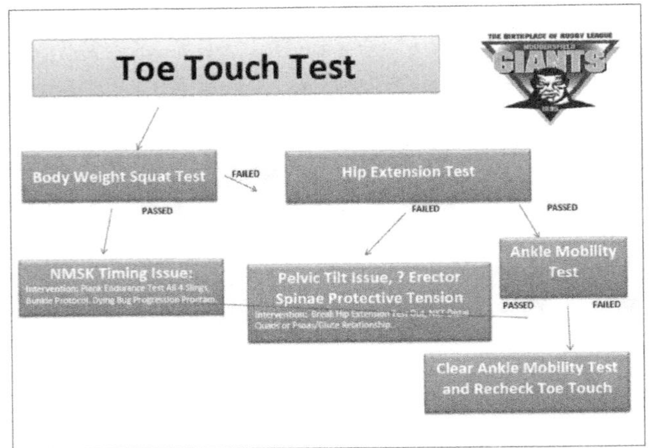

Here is an example of one of our clinical reasoning cross-reference sheets when we would cross-reference tests used to narrow down potential areas of perceived threat in combination with the athlete's injury history.

For the amateur sport healthcare professional, start small and focus on one or two things well and get confident at these before moving on to the next. If the reality of the situation is that you do not simply have enough staff or time to do everything above, start with pre-training markers and/or movements that will help give you baselines for potential injured joints later in the season and execute your movement prep sessions diligently using the principles outlined later.

It is the combination of the above that will help you prevent injuries and not one specific section but ACTION needs to be taken with the data which we will also discuss further in this book.

Summary of key points

The time spent screening should give you valuable information and data that can be used across the various parts of the machine. It is essential that the 'Go To' sports healthcare professional steps back, appreciates the athlete's nervous system has found value in self-organising the athlete in this way and can relate it back to the athlete's story.

To access a bonus webinar and further insight into my approach on movement screening visit: **www.injurypreventionbook.com/resources/**

CHAPTER 5

Pre-training markers micro system

Pre-training markers can be extremely useful to the 'Go To' sports healthcare professional. Now, if you recall, we have a structured and dedicated person every day to spend between 30 or 45 minutes absorbing, examining and reacting to the pre-training markers.

It is advisable to structure your pre-training markers so that your subjective wellness markers (looking at mood, sleep, appetite, muscle soreness/general aches and pains) are always done via an app ideally once the athlete wakes or is on the way into training and must be completed by a certain time. Our athletes usually completed theirs by 7.30am if the movement prep session started at 9am. This allowed us to catch signs of illness or athletes that may have some form of protective tone or may potentially not be training early that day. It also allowed my staff to make contact with athletes before they arrived and to arrange a suitable action plan in the form of liaising with the doctor, or the athlete coming into training earlier than usual so we could investigate the reason for this protective tone.

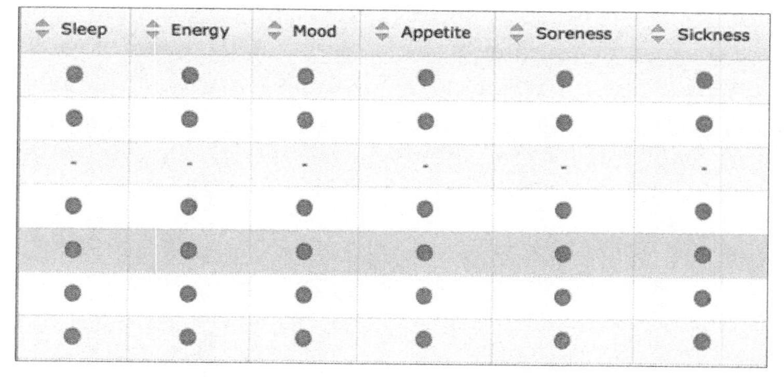

Sleep	Energy	Mood	Appetite	Soreness	Sickness
●	●	●	●	●	●
●	●	●	●	●	●
-	-	-	-	-	-
●	●	●	●	●	●
●	●	●	●	●	●
●	●	●	●	●	●
●	●	●	●	●	●

Here is an example of the subjective wellness report we would see every day at 7.30am on training days and slightly later at 11am on game days.

In my opinion, there is no point in doing the subjective wellness 30 minutes prior to training when there is very little time to even review the answers, let alone react appropriately.

This preliminary information gives us time to then discuss the findings with the strength and conditioning staff and/or with the head coaches if there is a trend across the board with the whole squad reporting unexpected findings. This helps you liaise early with coaches which will be important – this is discussed later in more detail. From experience, coaches don't like last-minute changes and will be quite reasonable if told about issues in advance, rather than landing the information on their table last minute.

When the athletes arrive at the training complex, they will then complete their objective markers upon arrival. This would usually need to be completed by 8.30am, 30 minutes prior to starting the movement prep session at 9am, for example. That gives you enough time to get the majority of the squad looked after. Then, if any problems do come up, you know who to prioritise and who to get your hands on. You can then assess the system's ability to self-organise and why there is, for example, a reduced range of movement on this particular day.

In recent years with the teams I consult with, I strongly recommend putting in a 3–4 minute pre-objective markers' mobility routine that entails the athletes quickly going over and under hurdles and some exercises designed to increase the lengthening ability of the diaphragm and encourage ribcage depression for 1–2 sets to decrease any stiffness that athletes might have from sleeping or travelling in the car. This will then help clear this up and we get a clearer picture in my opinion of true 'protective responses' that the nervous system may have laid from the previous day's training.

Ankle				Shoulder				Adductor		Toe-touch	
L	B	R	B	L	B	R	B		B		B
11	7	15	8	55°	40°	55°	40°	240	200	3	-7
12	12	13	12	70°	70°	↓ 70°	80°	240	170	↓ 0	1
0	10	0	10	0	50°	0	50°	0	220	0	1
11	11	↓ 11	12	50°	30°	60°	50°	240	235	↓ 0	3
↓ 10	11	↓ 9	12	↓ 55°	60°	↓ 55°	60°	280	270	↓ 0	2
10	9	10	8	70°	30°	60°	50°	↓ 280	295	↓ 1	3
↓ 10	11	↓ 9	11	↓ 25°	30°	↓ 20°	30°	170	170	2	1
16	15	10	10	32°	30°	32°	30°	220	220	-10	-10
0	8	0	4	0	50°	0	50°	0	280	0	2
↓ 7	8	↓ 5	8	↓ 50°	55°	50°	50°	↓ 160	250	↓ -3	-2
16	14	15	11	↓ 65°	70°	65°	60°	↓ 240	280	↓ 1	2
0	10	0	11	0	60°	0	50°	0	285	0	1
3	3	7	7	↓ 25°	30°	↓ 20°	30°	↓ 260	290	5	5
14	8	15	8	70°	60°	70°	55°	220	170	↓ 2	3

Here is an example of the pre-training marker scores we would see every day prior to training. Any players that were greater than 10% below baseline would be physically checked by the assistant therapist.

For the majority of athletes, a quick check and some directed movements for them should be enough to restore and reassure movement. If you feel that the athlete needs some help in restoring the range of movement, you could then do that through your focused hands-on treatment techniques but it is important to ensure that the athlete earns the right to restore the movement and create a long-lasting change in that range of movement for a specific movement in a specific direction.

The aim of the hands-on therapy intervention should ultimately be to decrease the perceived threat and restore and reassure their system that it is safe to produce force in specific directions. The athlete should be given some form of active movements that complement the treatment and further restore and reassure the system it is safe to put forces in specific directions, under even higher loads.

Just giving 'short-term' increases in range of motion through potentially reflexive means, without genuine exposure to loads in the directions where there is a perceived threat, is of limited value and can cause further negative reactions and muscle guarding, from my experience. The second episode of 'muscle guarding' or 'protective tone' that clinicians see on a daily basis can often be harder to 'undo' as the nervous system is potentially more sensitised now.

Ultimately, what you are doing with the pre-training markers is looking at how the body has set itself up in reaction to the previous day's training or previous day's load of that athlete.

If there are restrictions or reduced range of movements, the 'Go To' sports healthcare professional does not jump in and go, 'OK. He's got a tight calf or tight soleus', for example. They take into consideration what the athlete was doing the previous day. They understand the athlete's story and from there they can start to get a much better understanding of the primary stressors to this athlete. This, in combination with knowledge of the athlete's previous injuries (physical stressors), can then allow you to test the athlete's ability to self-organise by placing forces or perturbations to the athlete's particular tissues and see how he/she reacts.

In other words, what's NOT DOING ITS JOB that caused the soleus to potentially overwork in the first place? This is working smarter and not harder in my opinion.

We have a range of ways of assessing this that are taught in the ProSport Academy 'Go To' Therapist Mentorship, beyond the scope of this book. For more information on this, please visit: **www.thegotophysio.com/mentorship**

Using this approach, the 'Go To' Therapist is able to use this 30 to 45 minutes to find out directions of load tolerance that an athlete may be having trouble self-organising, restore and reassure the tissues lengthening capabilities locally, and then direct the athlete to one to two exercises to reassure their system that it is safe to load these tissues in a progressive graded exposure manner. The athlete will then go back and retest the range of motion.

If there is a general trend throughout the squad of reduced range of movement then this will be addressed as a group in your movement prep session and the programme design of this session will be adapted accordingly. The value of the Injury Prevention Machine is that you always have 15 minutes of movement prep time to react to what you are seeing as a group in pre-training markers and making informed clinical reasoning decisions of what to focus on in the movement prep sessions rather than just going through the motions.

You can change a lot in 15 minutes with movement if you give the body the right stimulus, and this should not be forgotten or dismissed. If you are in the middle of pre-season and a particularly higher load week, you should not be surprised to see a lot of red and orange pre-training marker scores (below 10-15% of pre-season screening baselines). This is the value in designing your Injury Prevention Machine in this way with the pre-training markers playing a big part in the movement prep design.

In my own Injury Prevention Machine, there was never a time where the pre-training markers across the board showed orange or red, then the athletes went straight into a field session. We always had the first 15 minutes of the day for our movement prep to restore and reassure range of motion. If on a particular day the athletes were going to the gym first, then the communication between the strength and conditioning coach and my team was absolutely essential. The strength and conditioning coach would then take this information and utilise it in their own warm-up in the gym sessions.

The 'Go To' sports professional understands the stress response as it applies to pre-training markers and is diligent in giving the athlete's system the correct stimulus to restore and reassure movement.

For example, using a standing toe touch test and understanding how the body reacts to stress can have new meaning. We can see that along an instantaneous axis or rotation when an athlete goes to touch their toes, one of the first tissues that is required to lengthen is the diaphragm's surrounding tissues as the ribcage depresses underneath.

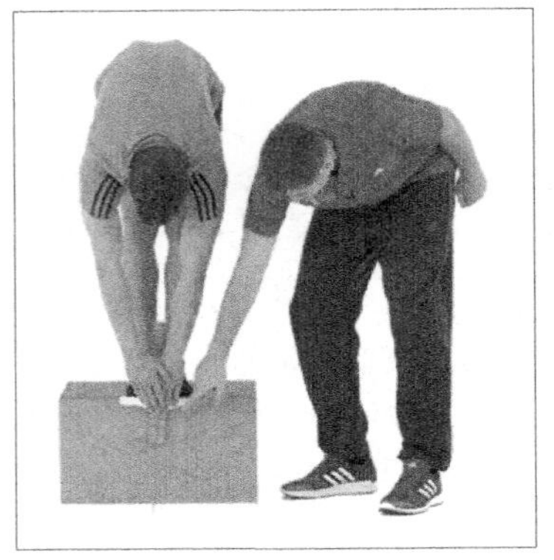

The toe touch test is so much more than hamstring length. It may also assess the ability of the ribcage to depress and the diaphragm to lengthen.

The 'Go To' Therapist can see from observing an athlete's stress response how valuable a standing toe touch test could be when an athlete is under loads and he is asked to subconsciously interact the systems and lengthen the diaphragm's surrounding tissues. An inability to touch the toes or have decreased range of movement scores on a particular day may not be indicative of 'tight hamstrings' but rather how the athlete's system has set itself up as a reaction to the day's previous stressors.

REST AND DIGEST
FIGHT OR FLIGHT REACTIONS
- Efortless/Easy Breathing
- Ability of Diaphram & Pelvic Floor to lengthen
- Confident 'Spring", 'Light' Movement Behaviour
- Awareness of Movement Patterns
- Clear Sensory Awareness of Body
- Movement Varability
- Good Weight Dstribution Through The Feet
- Controlled Breathing Through Movement
- Increased Breathing Rate & Depth
- Decreased Movement of Diaphragm & Pelvic Floor
- Protected Postures & Movement Patterns
- Decreased Awareness Or Recruitment
- 'Smudged' Motor Maps For Patterns of Movement
- Decreased Movement Varability
- Rigidity
- Poor Weight Distribution Through Feet
- Poor Control of Movement With the Breath

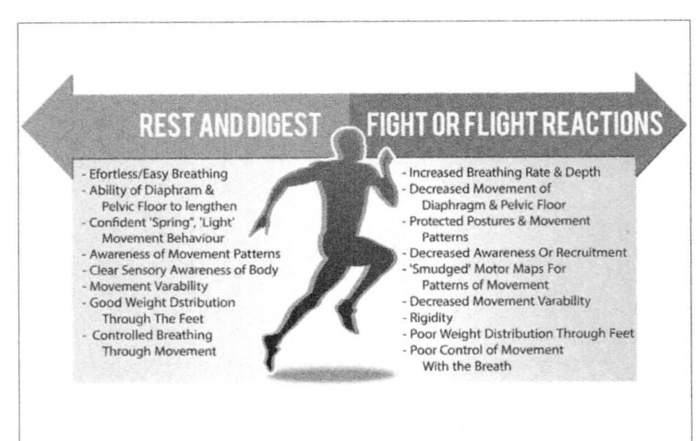

When an athlete is under extreme stress such as conditioning drills or contact, the body will be in predominantly sympathetic dominance which may have an impact on various other parts of the body.

If you recall in Chapter 2, the 'Go To' sports healthcare professional understands that when we go into fight or flight or extreme stress, we lose movement variability but we also lose movement ability of the diaphragm to lengthen. Recent studies show that increasing the diaphragm's range of movement can have an impact on the range of movement through tissues of the posterior chain and even neck range of motion. The whole body is connected and the 'Go To' Therapist appreciates this.

In my own Injury Prevention Machine, the standing toe touch test was used not as a hamstring length test but rather as a test to identify any athletes that may have self-organised into a common respiratory distress behavioural pattern. Rather than sending the athlete to get their hamstrings massaged to temporarily restore the ability to touch the toes and give a reflexive change, we would rather take a step back and ask ourselves how can we desensitise the respiratory system and improve the lengthening ability of the diaphragm which may have shortened or lost an ability to go through a full range of movement due to increased respiratory demands. If the diaphragm cannot lengthen, then the ribcage may struggle to depress, internally rotate and retract which may be contributing to a decreased toe touch or sit and reach scores.

Performing some basic respiratory desensitisation exercises and some specific hands-on treatment to facilitate this process can often instantaneously restore the range of motion required to perform the toe touch test and decrease the sensation of 'tightness' around the hamstrings, from my clinical experience.

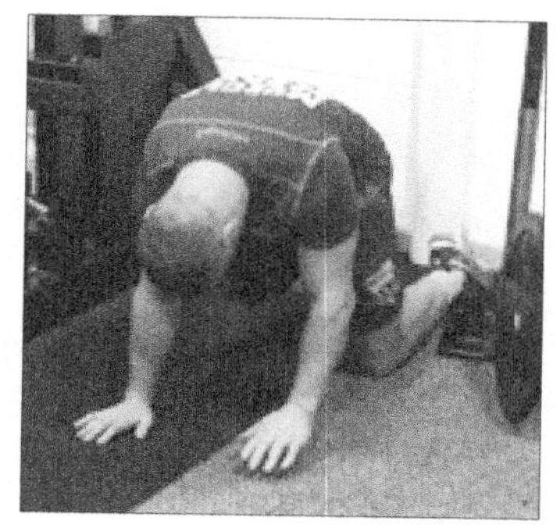

Here a player is performing an exercise to undo some of the sympathetic responses of the body and to mobilise the diaphragm while depressing the ribcage pre-training.

It is important, however, that the 'Go To' sports healthcare professional goes about reassuring and restoring the ability of all these tissues to interact together with the rest of the system such as the feet, the hands and other parts of the body in meaningful movements straight after, in an attempt to create long-lasting changes and not simple short-term changes.

I hope you consider value in how the 'Go To' sports healthcare professional looks at the body as one big system, understanding the reactions that happen to the body and not putting the musculoskeletal system and hamstring muscles on a pedestal in the above scenario, but addressing and asking the more intelligent question, 'Why are the tissues around the hamstrings actually holding this tone at the moment?' Is it because when the diaphragm gets hypertonic as a reaction to actual stress or perceived stress, the ribcage may lose the ability to mobilise? This could then potentially cause a prolonged lengthening effect on the tissues and the fascia surrounding the hamstrings which will be very rich in mechanoreceptors. These will be consistently communicating to the brain and could potentially be responsible for the sensation of tightness that the athlete is reporting. Just my thought process, anyway.

The intervention that the athlete receives may be completely different when the physio understands the stress responses of the body. Instead of giving them a 'hamstring stretch' or some form of intervention targeting the area that the athlete 'feels' is tight, the 'Go To' sports pro takes a step back and asks better questions. All of a sudden the intervention is completely different and is designed to restore the ability of the diaphragm and ribcage tissues to mobilise, shorten and lengthen again. And once we do this, we will see a completely different movement strategy that does not automatically direct forces to the hamstrings and gives the athlete much more movement options and variance of movement.

It is also the exact same with the knee to wall and shoulder rotation test. Although these tests were used, we would not make the assumption that just because an athlete had a decreased range of movement on the test it was down to a particular muscle or tissue. We would always trace it back to the stressor within the body. We would relate that to the player's subjective injury history for physical stressors and then we would test the athlete's ability to self-organise by applying a force in a specific direction and seeing how the athlete managed that load.

On occasions where there was a reduced motor output or a self-organising strategy that required a lot of excessive effort, we would then go about restoring and reassuring the system that it was indeed safe to put a load in this direction using some low load technique such as isometrics, and from there building up the load to ultimately reassure the system it was OK to move with thoughtless, fearless movement in a graded exposure manner.

If we could do that, we could then recheck the range of movement and very often the athlete's baseline pre-training markers would then have been restored. We have found this process to be much more valuable than simply assuming that just because an athlete has a decreased toe touch or sitting reach-out they need to stretch their hamstrings, or if an athlete has a decreased knee to wall that they need to lengthen the soleus tissues.

A better question for the 'Go To' sports pro to ask is why are the soleus tissues adapting with some form of protective tone? Understanding the athlete's injury history, their story and what they have done in the past few days are all major clues as to why these tissues may have adapted this way and, in the majority of cases, these tissues are doing a great job in the first place and are not just 'tight and weak'.

Understanding the tissue's axis rotation, understanding the direction of force, cross-referencing these tests with the athlete's subjective history and their pre-season screening information, and then further cross-referencing these tests with what the athlete has done the previous day can then allow us to make clinically reasoned decisions where we get the most bang for our buck in making quick but long-lasting changes to the pre-training markers.

I have found this approach to be the best use of my time over the last three years of working full-time in professional sport.

It can be extremely valuable to learn to ask better questions which ultimately allow you to see long-lasting changes in your athlete's pre-training markers rather than the athlete coming day in, day out with reduced range of movement. Once the athlete has earned the right to keep the range of movement through that graded exposure, then usually we will see these long-lasting changes.

The pre-training markers ultimately are to get a gauge and give us an insight into how the athlete's body has set itself up from the previous day's stressors, whether these were a result of training or other life events, and how they are managing today. Then from here, we're getting a gauge of what we need to include in the movement preparation sessions. Ideally, the majority of athletes would have restored their baseline markers prior to doing the movement prep. They would then have their 10-15 minutes movement prep session which would ultimately be dictated from that day's pre-training markers and the content in the session ahead so we could attempt to provide some form of graded exposure to the nervous system before they take to the field.

By now you should be able to clearly see the continuity of using our pre-season screening information and combining this with our pre-training markers which will then lead us nicely into implementing our movement preparation session.

Summary of key points

The pre-training markers should be viewed as a reaction of the body's ability to self-organise to the previous day's and week's load, both mentally and physically. The reactions we see from the athlete should be cross-referenced with their injury history and pre-season screening data along with an understanding of other potential stressors to their system to allow us to follow a logical step-by-step progression. Achieving long-lasting changes with pre-training markers should follow a continuum rather than just doing certain exercises and hoping something sticks.

CHAPTER 6

The pre-training movement preparation micro system

The old-school mentality of 'prehab' sessions of 10 minutes of foam rolling, some theraband exercises to 'strengthen' rotator cuff muscles and a few stretches is of limited value to the 'Go To' pro sports pro when we consider modern movement and pain science, in my opinion.

The aim of the pre-training movement preparation for the 'Go To' Therapist is threefold:

1. **To help us prepare the athlete's nervous system for the training session ahead to avoid any 'over-reactions' of the system by jumping, in load and speed of movement, too quickly on the field.**
2. **To help us restore and reassure the system to the previous day's 'over-reactions' as can be seen in the pre-training markers.**
3. **To help the athlete develop athleticism and be successful at absorbing and producing force as part of a more long-term athletic movement strategy in integration with the pre-season and in-season screening findings.**

The movement preparation micro system should be a continuum in your Injury Prevention Machine. Rather than just doing random exercises, the idea of the movement prep sessions should be to prepare the athlete for what's about to come today and to manage the reactions of yesterday first and foremost. In addition, helping an athlete manage their own body weight and the ground reaction forces applied to it in a variety of different directions is of much more value to the 'Go To' Therapist for the athlete than some isolated non-meaningful movements, in my experience.

A successful movement prep session is ultimately a graded exposure into the loads that are going to be placed upon the body in any given contact session or any given field session on this day. The actual execution of a successful movement prep session is to ensure that the athlete has the ability to shorten and lengthen tissues in any given direction, absorb forces and manage them well through their body so that they can overcome them and produce a reactive force in any given direction.

The pre-season screening, pre-training markers and daily markers will give the 'Go To' sports therapist a lot of valuable information regarding what tissues may be carrying protective tone.

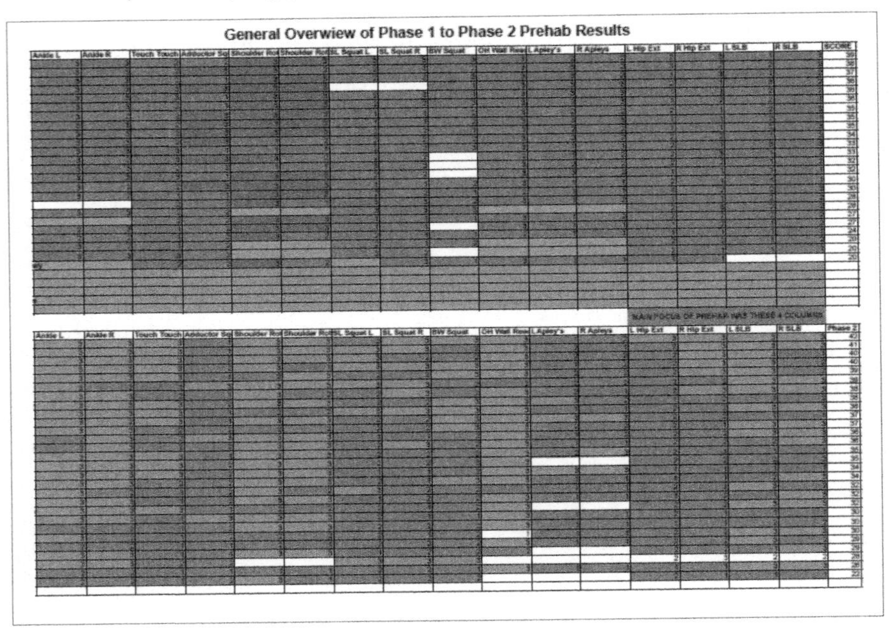

Here is an example of a spreadsheet after pre-season and in-season screening. The areas of red would help direct my attention to the types of movements that will help facilitate improvement in the squad's overall athleticism during the movement prep sessions.

In regards to the overall goal of improved athleticism, the 'Go To' Therapist is also exposing their athletes to a structured deceleration programme in a graded exposure manner so the athlete has an ability to absorb forces well under higher loads before they go into their actual on-field sessions.

Practically, from my own past experiences, pre-season was usually about restoring length through the diaphragm and pelvic floor tissues and ultimately undoing sympathetic stress reactions on the body while putting the starting foundations of the deceleration programme in place. In-season, as the training loads decreased dramatically and intensity increased, was more about restoring the range of motion to peripheral tissues, and managing and absorbing forces well with the higher level progressions in the deceleration programme.

Giants Movement Preparation 2012/2013

PHASE 1 Weeks 1-3

Movement [illegible]	[illegible]	[illegible]	[illegible]	[illegible]	[illegible]	[illegible]
Postural Restoration Exercise 1-2	10 Mins	√				
Postural Restoration Exercise 3-4	10 Mins	√				
Hurdles	4 Mins	Sprinter Arms Front Leg Flexn, Back Leg Internal Rotn.	Backward with Hip Internal Rotn Superslow	Lateral Lunge Glides	Sprinter Arms Front Leg Flexn, Back Leg Internal Rotn.	Lateral Lunge Glides
Glute/Traps Activation	4 Mins			Band Walks Monster Walks Linear	Band Walks Lateral	Band Duck Walks
Hopping Linear/ Lateral / Rotational	4 Mins	Linear	Lateral	Linear		Rotational Phase 1 (0-45 Degrees)
T Spine with Hips	4 Mins	Sumo Squat with Macarena	Muslim Pray Cat Camel with Hip Extensions	Sumo Squat with Macarena	Muslim Pray Cat Camel with Hip Extensions	Worlds Greatest Stretch
Isolated Muscle Stretch	4 Mins	V Quads with Pec Stick Stretch Off Wall / Flexor Pumps	Sidelying Quad Stretch with Flexor Pumps	Pec Major and Minor Stretch Off Floor	Sidelying Quad Stretch with Flexor Pumps	Quad With Stick Pec Stretch Flexor Pumps
Core	4 Mins		Dying Bug + Leg Drops with Wall		Bridge with Leg Extension Test	

Here is an example of a Movement Prep document I used in 2013 during phase 1 of the movement prep. This was the result of taking into account the athlete's injury history, the pre-season screen and the content coming up during phase 1 of pre-season training.

In a nutshell, the strength and conditioning coach and the coaches would ultimately stress the athlete to the nth degree and take them to a 'dark place' in pre-season. The 'Go To' Therapist would ask the intelligent question: 'What is this athlete's subconscious mind thinking about this stress right now and what measures is he/she putting in place to make him/her successful or to just get through this?'

The next day in pre-season would ultimately be focused on restoring and reassuring the lengthening of the diaphragm, restoring movement options, restoring the ability of the tissues to shorten and lengthen and reassuring the body to absorb forces well in a variety of different directions. Then the athletes would be sent off down to the field for a prolonged running session, into a high intensity contact session or into the gym for an almost maximal loading weight session and the cycle of protective strategies would start all over again.

The reality is that's what happens in pre-season training. For me to be obsessed with my pre-season markers and trying to improve movement screens from two to three, etc. may not be realistic during these six weeks or so.

If I can break through pre-season without any soft tissue injuries and the athlete has the same movement screen 'scores' then I'm happy. I would take that any day over picking up two or three hamstring, groin or cuff injuries, but improving my movement screening scores by one or two and my excel spreadsheet looking a bit more green or orange. I hope this is beginning to make sense and you can appreciate the realities of sport and the challenges you will be faced with in the real world.

Overall, in pre-season, I would very much be looking at the athlete's stress responses, both physically and mentally, to the loads and how they are coping with these.

A key section of my movement screen would be restoring the ability of the diaphragm and pelvic floor to lengthen and shorten which in effect would help the thoracic spine which would help pelvic mobility and restore movement options. From there, it's about restoring and reassuring the lengthening of the tissues whether that's skin, fascia, nerves, arteries, veins or muscles and then applying forces in specific directions in reaction to any various perturbations to restore movement variability and stability reflexively.

The pre-movement prep sessions would usually start with some form of a drill where we need to ensure that the athlete is exhaling for a prolonged period in order to lengthen the diaphragm maximally. From there, we may do some form of movement that requires the full body to interact and that uses the tissues we have already identified as needing to lengthen and shorten under control with externally focused tasks. Towards the back end of the movement prep session, we may have some form of graded exposure deceleration programme to the types of movements that the athlete is about to undergo in the session ahead.

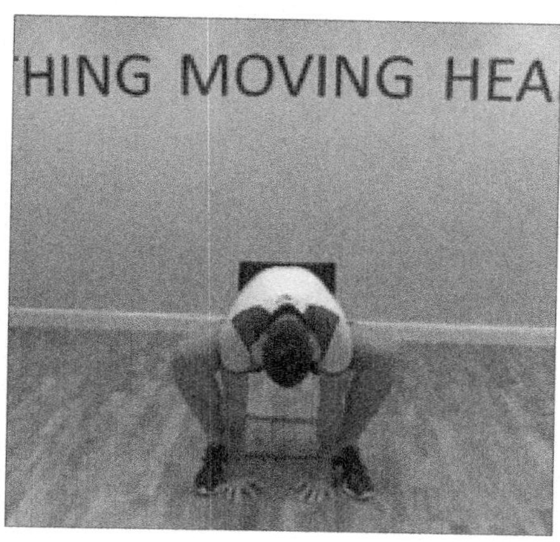

Here is a movement I used a lot during the 2017 Rugby League World Cup in Australia pre-training to help mobilise the diaphragm and pelvic floor.

The first few weeks in a movement prep session I am more focused on the athlete absorbing forces in a very much lower level to avoid causing protective reactions. The 'Go To' Therapist understands that the athlete needs to earn the right to progress and simply going to the higher loading 'sexier' deceleration drills may encourage higher threshold movement strategies and potential negative motor adaptations from the nervous system.

As we progress through pre-season, we may then apply more loads on the athlete in the form of some structured deceleration progressions where we increase load and speed of movement. Again, the athletes need to earn the right to get to the 'higher load' drills.

The first couple of weeks may be all about an athlete learning to absorb forces in movements such as lunges, progressing to some form of a hop and a stick type movement whereas towards the end of pre-season, we may then be concentrating on some actual acceleration and deceleration drills asking the athlete to stop in a particular time under higher ground reaction forces, observing forces well through the system and not through one particular joint or particular high threshold movement strategy.

Executing your movement prep session

In regards to organising your movement preparation, it is essential that you have a session that lasts 10-12 minutes, potentially all the way up to 15 where athletes are engaged and not standing around and getting distracted.

From experience, if the athletes are standing still or doing something that is not stimulating enough, what will happen is the players will start chatting, the quality of the session will go down, the therapist will get frustrated and ultimately it will be a waste of time.

The secret to combating this problem is all in the set-up of your session.

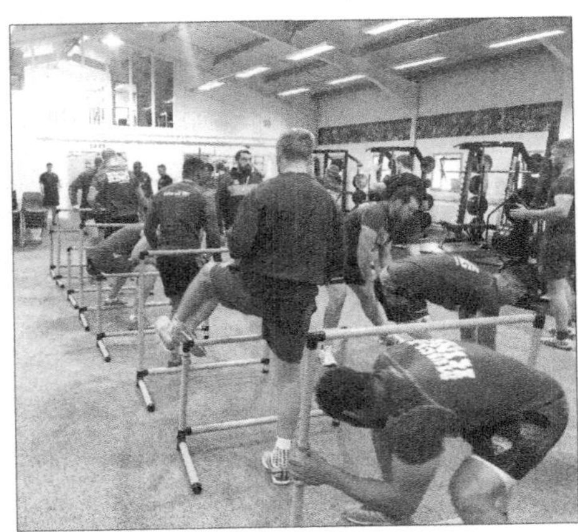

Here are the Giants performing a pre-training movement prep session in 2015.

If you have a $20m^2$ space then you have enough room to successfully perform a movement prep session successfully with 30 athletes.

The room would ultimately be set up like a track where the athlete starts at one corner and goes up one lane performing some form of dynamic movement and comes down the next performing some different variation, and so on, until they have been up and down each lane using different exercises.

The exercise choice needs to be dynamic; it needs to flow, but it needs to serve a particular purpose. The placement of exercises in particular lanes also needs to be taken into account. If one particular exercise is able to be executed rather quickly and then the next lane coming down are taking longer to perform another movement, this may cause the line to slow and create a backlog of players at one end of the room. This again leads to chatting and disengaged athletes.

To see a real-life example of one of my previous movement preparation sessions, please visit **www.injurypreventionbook.com/resources**

Unfortunately, getting this right comes with experience, but you need to be able to adjust and figure out on the go which exercise you put after which exercise. This would be the strategy I would opt for to make a system flow and be more dynamic. However, the quality in the execution of the exercises goes down slightly as there is less time for coaching of the movements. Therefore, I prefer to use this type of set-up in-season if possible once the athletes are familiar with the movements and are able to execute good movement qualities.

If you need more quality coaching opportunities such as the first time you are introducing certain movements to the group, another option is to have your athletes split into no more than four to five players per group and spend five minutes per station or three minutes per station, working with one therapist. The obvious downfall of this is, the more groups you have, the more therapists you will need.

As a compromise, I've always found if we can start the session with the athletes doing the first one or two exercises all together as a group and in a static position, this allows you to quickly screen for the elephants in the room who need a little more coaching and then from here go into the lane-type drills.

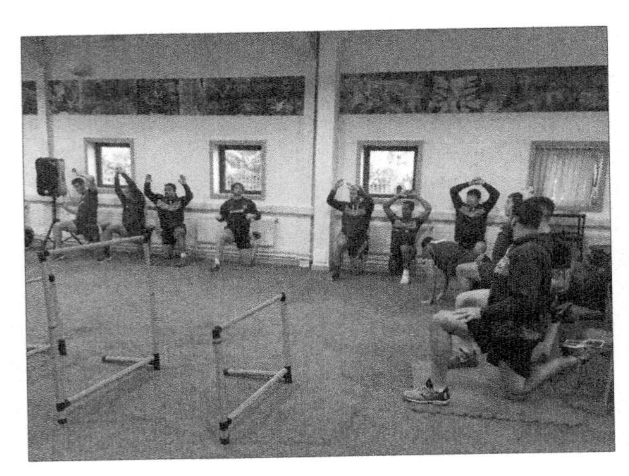

Team starting movement prep with group 3 dimensional lengthening of the quadriceps identified as being required from the pre-season and in-season movement screens.

The first one or two exercises may be a diaphragm or pelvic floor lengthening and shortening drill, designed to restore the ability of these to lengthen and shorten as well as one other exercise you've identified from your pre-training markers that is important to do well. From here, once we ensure that the athletes have all performed the most important movements to attack the pre-training markers, they can then go to the lanes to perform more dynamic meaningful movements.

Timing your sessions

In pre-season, I would be happy to spend a full 15 minutes that would have been allocated to 'movement prep' in order to restore lengthening because it may be needed due to excessive loads and hence excessive reactions on the athlete's body. Once we got to in-season, I would need less time to restore and reassure these reactions and my movement prep sessions were more focused on the drills that were about to happen that day and aiming to give the athlete some form of graded exposure stimulus they were about to go under on the field.

If the team or squad were in a de-load week, I would try my best to replicate my movement prep session with the rest of the coaching staff so that everything was short and sharp, so it fed in nicely to what the strength and conditioning coaches and head coaches were trying to achieve that week.

Although the duration decreased and the intensity may have increased, the quality of the sessions never suffered.

The continuum needs to be from the therapist to the conditioner to the coach with all on the same wavelength in order for this to be a fully successful injury prevention system, in my opinion.

Your movement prep sessions prior to gym sessions may also be aimed at improving an athlete's ability to be more successful with their lifts or movements in the gym but for me having a movement prep session prior to going to the field was non-negotiable.

The pre-training markers and movement preparation sessions can work really well if executed well and the players buy into it. We personally got great results when doing it this way, setting it up so that over time we had a broad plan: we knew where we were trying to get to, we were progressing the athletes systematically every two weeks with our exercise design, but the underlying foundations and the intentions always remained the same, working towards the long-term plan of athletic ability.

Summary of key points

The movement preparation session should be used to help restore and reassure the 'reactions' to how the athlete self-organised themselves from the previous day's and week's sessions. It should have a clear goal of restoring and reassuring the tissues' ability to shorten and lengthen, absorb and produce force in multiple directions and help the athlete become exposed gradually to the load demands that will be placed upon their systems on any particular day. The practical execution of the actual session is important to consider, to ensure the athletes are engaged and executing the movements well.

CHAPTER 7

The on-feet loading micro system

A very important facet of the injury prevention system is the monitoring and adaptation of time on feet. Having a coach who is aware of the impact of time on feet that the athletes undergo on a daily basis is important. Working with a good coach who appreciates that they need to stick to a certain time on feet each day can provide massive help to your own injury prevention system.

And this comes down to three important facets that are also overlooked:

1. **The interaction between the head coach and the performance team.**
2. **The relationship between the strength and conditioning coach and the medical department.**
3. **The ability to use meaningful information and be proactive without overreacting using the data to logically inform the coach of the reason WHY you are asking to adapt, reduce or increase the load on a particular day.**

From my experience, what really differentiates the best head strength and conditioning coach or head of performance coach is the ability to 'manage' the head coach with regards time on feet.

In order for the 'time on feet' management to be successful, and before we even discuss the scientific research and 'ideals', the strength and conditioning coach and the physiotherapist need to be on the same page and communicating the same key message to the coach on a daily basis.

There certainly is strength in numbers and the message needs to be communicated well from all parties sometimes in order for the coaching staff to actually listen.

The following is an example of how this has worked previously with the Huddersfield Giants. The Head of Strength and Conditioning at the time, Greg Brown, would note the GPS loads were higher than anticipated. My team would notice that the pre-training markers were particularly red when we had not particularly planned for this and there was a very big day ahead. Greg would then usually approach me prior to seeing the head coach and let me know his information and I would communicate mine so that we would be on the same wavelength in the message that we were communicating to the coach.

Now, we were not trying to manipulate the coach but were simply making sure that if the medical department and the performance department were giving the same message, and the head coach decided to override them both and to go ahead as planned without some form of modification, then he/she would ultimately have to accept the consequences of this decision if there were any injuries or issues from the session. To a point, the head coach is not interested in stats and figures but can clearly see how having two or three of their best players on the sidelines and missing six weeks of pre-season has potential consequences on their ability to perform their job well.

The visual reminder of red or green can be particularly useful in helping the coach to logically understand the WHY. The reality is they don't care about 10% of baselines being down and just want to coach. However if they see a whole host of red across the page for the baselines then most coaches can appreciate that there is a general reaction from the squad and action may need to be taken. This was certainly my experience.

Ankle				Shoulder				Adductor		Toe-touch	
L	B	R	B	L	B	R	B		B		B
11	7	15	8	55°	40°	55°	40°	240	200	3	-7
12	12	13	12	70°	70°	↓ 70°	80°	240	170	↓ 0	1
0	10	0	10	0	50°	0	50°	0	220	0	1
11	11	↓ 11	12	50°	30°	60°	50°	240	235	↓ 0	3
↓ 10	11	↓ 9	12	↓ 55°	60°	↓ 55°	60°	280	270	↓ 0	2
10	9	10	8	70°	30°	60°	50°	↓ 280	295	↓ 1	3
↓ 10	11	↓ 9	11	↓ 25°	30°	↓ 20°	30°	170	170	2	1
16	15	10	10	32°	30°	32°	30°	220	220	-10	-10
0	8	0	4	0	50°	0	50°	0	280	0	2
↓ 7	8	↓ 6	8	↓ 50°	55°	50°	50°	↓ 160	250	↓ -3	-2
16	14	15	11	↓ 65°	70°	65°	60°	↓ 240	280	↓ 1	2
0	10	0	11	0	60°	0	50°	0	285	0	1
3	3	7	7	↓ 25°	30°	↓ 20°	30°	↓ 260	290	5	5
14	8	15	8	70°	60°	70°	55°	220	170	↓ 2	3

It is common to see 3-4 reds on a day-to-day basis with the team's objective markers. During pre-season you may see the majority of the screen red which is fine if it was previously planned to be a big day; the movement prep can be adjusted today accordingly. The problem arises when there is a lot of red and it was not planned to have been a taxing day on the athlete's nervous system. This is then where effective communication between medical, performance and coaching staff is essential.

I hope you can now see why it is essential that the strength and conditioning coach and the head physiotherapist have a very good working relationship with the ultimate mutual goals of both being there for the benefit and health care of the athletes.

It is essential that the coach follows a structured time frame of time on feet as directed by the strength and conditioning department but ultimately as part of an overall periodised programme. A coach who will stick to the time frames allotted and won't go over 5–10 minutes every session will have a massive effect on your ability to control your injury prevention system from my experience.

The majority of on-feet loading will be monitored from the strength and conditioning department as this will need to take into account all facets from gym loads to on-feet running loads to contact loads.

The final component to the on-feet loading is to understand that sometimes just because a squad's GPS loads are higher than anticipated or the pre-training markers are redder than anticipated, we need to make a common sense and logical call. Shielding athletes too much may not actually help them in the long-term. Tim Gabbett's research is a great example of this in how the acute to chronic workload ratios are important to understand.

The athletes need to train hard and have tolerance to load in order to become robust and resilient; however it is a fine line. From a medical point of view, it is worth being familiar with Tim's work. He has some great 'real world' ways of monitoring the acute to chronic workload ratios to avoid any spikes in training loads.

Tim's research is readily available online and although there may be some questions surrounding the exact robustness of the acute:chronic workload to injury prediction, in my opinion it is still better than not monitoring training loads at all and can easily be implemented in the real world, which is very attractive to me personally.

Change of surfaces

Another scenario that the 'Go To' Therapist needs to be careful with is the football coach wanting to change surfaces often. Once the ground is heavy, the quality of the skills sessions may suffer so the natural tendency for some coaches is to use alternative surfaces such as 3G surfaces.

While there are some research papers looking at this and more information will presumably become clear (or not) on the impact of surfaces such as 3G on injury rates in the future, the 'Go To' sports therapist will take a step back and ask themselves some questions to help gain an insight into why some athletes' old niggles tend to flare up on these surfaces.

If there is one thing I know to be true it is that human beings in general do not like change. A change in surface and potentially increased ground reaction forces combined with an athlete's lack of readiness for such loading could potentially cause old nociceptors to go from a refractory state to a more active state and contribute to this pain output or reactions that the athlete is now experiencing.

Personally, I do not fear surfaces such as 3G for my athletes once I know that the athletes have a good ability to absorb forces well and have been exposed to these in the movement prep sessions in the weeks beforehand but also in the session on this particular day. If the athletes are training on such surfaces, a graded exposure warm-up may be beneficial in the form of additional deceleration work prior to the session starting on this surface. This may help potentially desensitise the peripheral tissues to such loads so the athlete does not go from an 'all from nothing' approach with the first few decelerations in the skills sessions.

The 'Bayesian Brain' and the predictive processing model really interest me in regards the reactions we see from athletes when they change surfaces. Could the errors perceived in ground reaction forces absorbed from athletes lead to increased prediction errors transmitting to the higher centres of the brain that leads to the athlete experiencing a conscious experience of old injuries becoming grumpy?

If we use our movement prep time or warm-up time pre-session on this particular surface and allow the athlete to update their belief system and perception on ground reaction forces through a graded exposure to deceleration drills, could this lead to a decrease in prediction errors and less reactions such as pain, swelling or muscle guarding post-session? This is obviously just my thoughts but I think this may potentially have something to do with the positive results we have seen when using this approach pre-training when having to change surface.

An athlete who can absorb forces well in three planes of motion to the necessary higher loads, transfer forces well through the hamstrings to the hip and from the gastrocnemius down to the Achilles tendon should have nothing to fear about training on such surfaces; it is the 'Go To' Therapist's job to ensure that the movement prep sessions are helping the athlete achieve this in addition to the work done by the strength and conditioning coach.

For more information on predictive processing, I recommend the work of Andy Clark, Jacob Hohwy and more recently Mick Thacker, of whom I await the outcome of his next PhD papers with great interest.

Summary of key points

It is important that there is a mutually respectful relationship between the head coach, the performance department and the medical department. The medical and performance departments should in particular have a great working relationship and be able to pick up on the same stress reactions from the body via their own individual monitoring systems that they are using. Time on feet and also changing surfaces should be monitored closely but ultimately it comes down to how well the athletes are prepared and how robust they are to cope with the demands of their working environment.

CHAPTER 8

Moving well under heavy loads micro system

Move well in the gym; move well on the field…

That is what I believe and I continue to use in my lectures. Having that kind of mindset from a physiotherapist point of view can then justify why you should have a presence in the gym and appreciate the importance of strength training.

One of the best things Meirion Jones (my own original mentor) and I did in 2008–2009 with Leeds Rhinos was to actually be in the gym with the players while they were lifting. Now you need to understand your place and have a good relationship with your strength and conditioning coach with the sole purpose of actually helping them coach the players, which I think is massively overlooked these days.

Now, it can be quite frustrating at times because you seem to be consistently saying the same cues and same messages to the players yet they will always tend to go back to their usual high threshold strategies. With that said, the ability to educate players on correct foot pressures, distributing weight well through the full foot, lifting well under high loads and also pulling and rowing well will result in massive rewards for the medical department from my experience.

We certainly saw our soft tissue injuries rate dramatically reduce in the 2008-2009 season and this was a big factor in my opinion in having a fully fit squad for the grand final. This, combined with the later years of structuring our pre-season screening and movement prep sessions in a systematic way, can really multiply the effectiveness of the injury prevention system presented in this book.

Before we look at what lifting well in the gym looks like, let's take a look at how the 'Go To' sports therapist might appreciate reactions that happen in the body as a result of not lifting well in the gym and how it might impact the ability to execute an effective Injury Prevention Machine.

A common reaction that is seen with athletes under higher loads is to maintain all the weight through a specific portion of the foot (usually either the heels or the opposite end of the foot, the toes).

I personally believe the cue of 'push through your heels' or similar cues are causing a lot of issues for athletes. We only have to appreciate the gait cycle and the self-organising strategy that the body adopts to utilise elastic energy to appreciate the importance of each part of the body and in particular the full foot doing its job.

When the weight is on the heel during the gait cycle, this couples with the hip in flexion but when the hip is extending, this usually couples with the weight going through the midfoot. At the end of the push-off the weight is on the toes at the end of the hip extension.

Therefore, if the body self-organises this way, there must be some merit in these parts of the foot coupling with the hip movement for optimal management of ground reaction forces. Managing these forces throughout the body to utilise elastic energy to recoil back into the ground is a magnificent achievement that I think we need to be encouraging in the gym also.

Another method worth studying is the foot pressure during the Olympic lifting movements; the ability to organise the body and external loads to lift with such speed and power is magnificent to observe. Again you will notice the hip is in flexion when the weight is in the heels during these specific lifts and as the hip extends, the weight distribution is transferring towards the mid- and front foot.

In fact, just prior to the most explosive part of the Olympic lifting movement, the second pull, the weight is on the midfoot, which makes sense when you think about the midfoot giving the athlete an ability to utilise all the muscles in the lower limb. If they use the heel instead they may lose the ability to plantarflex efficiently through the ankle joint which will affect the lower leg muscles, distal hamstrings and possibly the glutes.

I believe when athletes are lifting in the gym, the same weight distributions should follow gait or Olympic lifting to encourage movement variability and help the self-organising ability of the nervous system for optimal movement efficiency as can be seen during Olympic lifting.

However, from my own experience this coupling of efficient foot pressures and hip movements can often get mismanaged under higher loads and cued ineffectively by the strength and conditioning or medical professional.

The two strategies that will usually follow are:

1 **Weight on the toes as the hip goes into flexion**

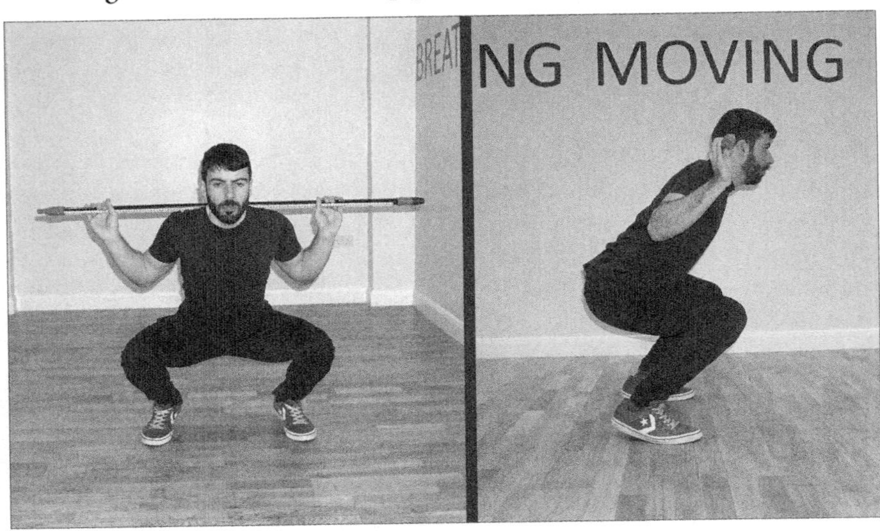

Notice the weight is excessively on the toes. The weight shift forward will cause the low back and knees to do work at the beginning of the ascent instead of the knees, delaying knee extension and allowing the hips to do more work.

From my experience, this will usually result in excessive forward-travelling knees, limit true hip flexion and increase the forward lean of the torso with the lumbar extensors having to react to maintain balance. This makes it difficult for the hamstrings to co-contract at the knee, with the quadriceps and soleus doing most of the work with the lumbar extensors. The lower back will also have to counteract the forwards foot pressure to actually prevent the athlete from moving forwards.

If this athlete presents with knee or back pain, is it the patella tendon's fault or the SI joint's fault that they become irritated? Will performing isometrics for the tendon or even eccentrics help if the athlete returns to the gym and continues to lift like this?

2. **Weight on the heels as the hips go into extension**

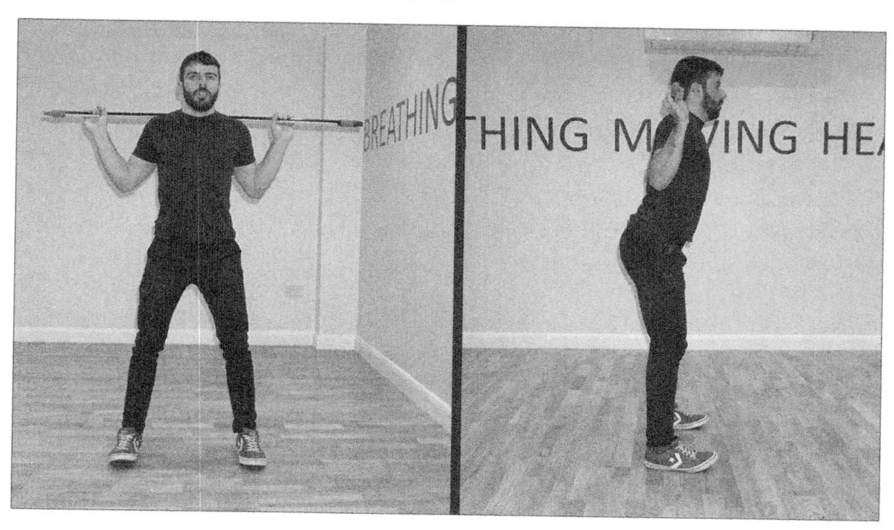

Notice the athlete starts with the weight on the heels. This causes a reaction of excessive protraction of the ribcage forward to balance which will increase lumbar extensor activity while also decreasing the ability to plantarflex the feet and utilise the distal hamstrings and proximal gastrocnemius which will be important to utilise through the ascent back up.

In an attempt to solve the knees going too far forwards, in the early 2000s the cue of keeping the weight through the heels became popular and this is the more common problem I see nowadays.

The majority of athletes are starting the lift with all the weight on their heels and this results in a lack of weight distribution through the full foot. This affects the ability of the distal hamstrings and proximal gastrocnemius to co-contract at the knee efficiently and to allow the hip joint to do genuine work due to a lack of plantar flexion forces and an inability to delay knee extension via a co-contraction at the knee joint. The quadriceps now tend to do excessive work and the knees 'snap back' with the low back then having to hyper extend at the top of the lift and the athlete consciously squeezes the glutes.

Check this out for yourself, even in a seated position, push through the heels while placing one hand under the distal hamstring on one side and the other on the proximal fibres of the glute max with the other. You more than likely will feel little activity. Now push through the midfoot to forefoot as if squashing an orange through the floor while keeping the hands in the same positions. You should hopefully feel more distal hamstrings and gastrocnemius contributing to the movement and then a reaction slightly delayed through the glute max.

Would you rather an athlete distribute the load evenly through the whole limb or use excessive muscles and joints to compensate for other tissues not doing their jobs?

If the athlete is coached to push through the heels mainly through the ascent, it is then common to see the lower back arching at the top of the lift and the athlete having to consciously 'squeeze the glutes'. It is difficult to engage the proximal fibres of gluteus maximus consciously while the weight is on the heels. Give it a go. Now repeat while the weight is on the midfoot going towards the forefoot.

If the weight distribution travels forward towards the midfoot as the hip extends, you will naturally feel the proximal glutes engage during mid-stance and, more importantly, the distal hamstrings will continue to engage throughout the movement, similar to the sequencing we require when sprinting.

If the weight stays on the heel, I usually see athletes snap the knee back with the quads and overarch the back in order to return to the start position.

The weight needs to start through the midfoot and then travel towards the heels as the hip goes into flexion so that the weight distribution goes towards the midfoot as the hip extends. This allows an opportunity for the athlete to manage perturbatory loads subconsciously and manage their base of support. It will also utilise the distal hamstrings and proximal gastrocnemius and promote a more efficient co-contraction at the knee joint, delaying knee extension so the hip joint can do more work.

If we have athletes who present with proximal hamstring issues or patellofemoral pain, or the lower back continues to become irritated, will performing isometrics for the tendon and even eccentrics help if the athlete returns to the gym and continues to lift like this?

In both cases above, the 'Go To' Therapist appreciates that if the athlete continues to lift like this under higher loads, certain tissues are becoming excessively loaded and ultimately over time may become sensitised, which may result in subtle interactions, as the work of Kylie Tucker, Paul Hodges and colleagues have shown.

We may then see further alterations in the athlete's movement strategies and the injury that eventually presents in the form of a tendon or muscle injury may be a further reaction. I appreciate there is a lot of theory here, but I'd just like to share my thought process.

For a practical demonstration of what I mean in these two strategies and the importance of ensuring good foot pressures please visit **www.injurypreventionbook.com/resources**

Therefore the Injury Prevention Machine ensures that all bolts are securely tightened and doesn't allow one joint to take excessive strain on the whole machine. Getting the athlete lifting well in the lifts below is essential in order to reduce nociceptors becoming active, contributing to alterations in movement strategies that ultimately may lead to actual tissue injury.

I hope you can see the value in investing in the athlete lifting well through a full range of movement and helping the strength and conditioning department in achieving this with your movement preparation programme and soft tissue prescription in reaction to your movement screen. In my opinion, there is no point in executing a very good pre-season screening, a very good movement prep session if the athlete when under high loads tends to lift in suboptimal manners that will contribute towards nociceptors becoming potentially grumpy and contributing to the reactions that may follow. This may be the athlete presenting to you with Achilles issues, patellar tendon issues, shoulder issues, etc.

The 'Go To' Therapist will ask better questions though. Is it because of weak rotator cuff muscles or weak glutes? Or is it simply because that was this athlete's strategy to handle this load and the stress around the system that has ultimately caused the athlete to come to you further down the line with this acute injury. Is the rotator cuff weak and painful because it was weak in the first place or was it because it was directing a lot of traffic that eventually caused it to become weak and painful? Was it the Achilles' fault or due to a weak gastrocnemius muscle or maybe the gastrocnemius was doing a great job directing the force down to the Achilles due to excessive pressure on the front of the foot when doing all the lifts and when decelerating?

Again I wish it was as easy as these scenarios but the 'Go To' sports therapist needs to be asking these questions.

Other common high threshold strategies I see for specific lifts are covered on the following pages.

Deadlift

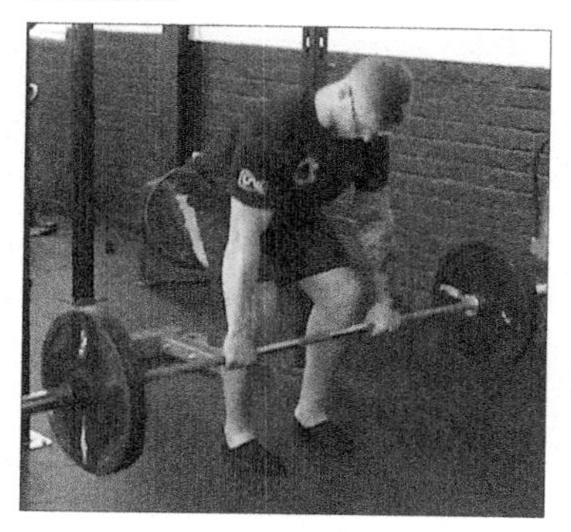

The start position of the deadlift needs to have intent through the midfoot to overcome all slack in the hamstrings prior to the ascent. As the bar comes up and the hips go into extension, there needs to be a genuine extension of the hips travelling horizontally over the midfoot towards the forefoot.

The deadlift start position is usually performed incorrectly among Rugby Union or Rugby League players. I rarely see players take up the slack in the hamstrings before initiating the lift. A lack of intent through the midfoot and too much weight on the heels will result in this, from my experience.

Athletes usually tend to set themselves up with the weight too far back on the heels. This usually results in the athlete directing a lot of force through the proximal hamstrings and through the SI joint / thoracic lumbar fascia resulting in protective tension or tone through the lower back area due to not enough help from the gastrocnemius and distal hamstrings to allow forces to be directed through the knee joint and the hip from the ground.

An intent of squashing an orange through the midfoot while some weight is on the heels prior to lifting the bar will actually result in the hips going higher than the knees, slack being taken out of the hamstrings and a much more efficient strategy is in place to distribute the load throughout the body. This will also help the midfoot contribute while the hip is extending, rather than extending the hips with the weight on the heels. Give both versions a try and notice the differences.

Bent-over row

The bent-over row also tends to have the same issue where the full slack is not overcome in the hamstrings; therefore, the system is not in the stable position to handle the load directed during dynamic movement of the barbell in a bent-over row position.

The risk reward of these movements is questionable; however, what's of more importance is that if these movements are included in your athlete's strength and conditioning programme, you educate them on how to take up the slack in the hamstrings at the starting position.

An intent of squashing an orange through the midfoot while some weight is on the heels prior to lifting the bar will actually result in the hips going higher than the knees, slack being taken out of the hamstrings and a much more efficient strategy will be in place to distribute the load throughout the body and to engage the proximal glutes more fully.

Romanian deadlift

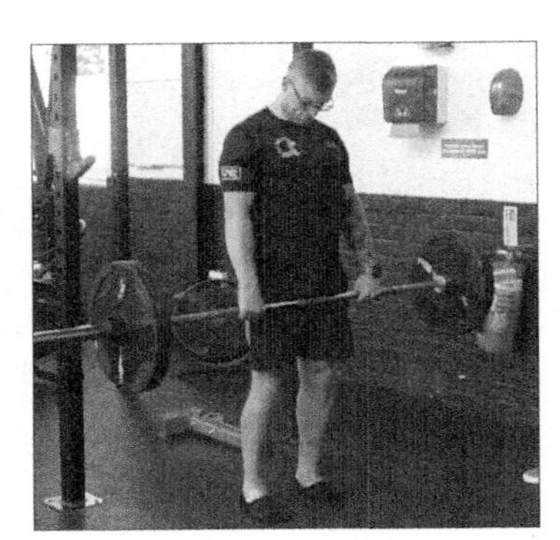

The RDL start position should be with the weight through the midfoot. As the bar descends, the weight should travel towards the heel while maintaining some pressure through midfoot and forefoot for balance.

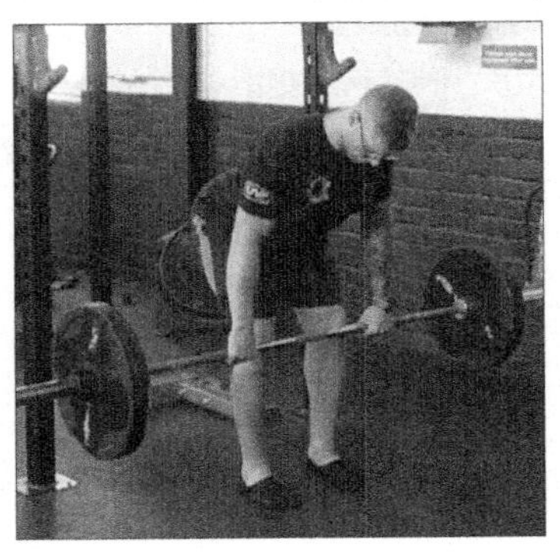

As the bar ascends in the RDL movement, the hips need to have genuine intent in travelling horizontally over the midfoot with the knees still slightly flexed. An incorrect movement would be no horizontal motion of the hips and the knees snapping backwards with an excessive overarching of the lower back.

One of the biggest errors I see with a Romanian deadlift is an athlete again not taking up the slack in the hamstrings or a lack of movement through the foot during this lift. As the load increases, the athlete will tend to manage this external load usually with excessive pressure on the toes or on the heels but will be unable to display good weight distribution through the foot during the hip flexion and extension.

Most athletes will start with the weight on the heels which makes it difficult to distribute more weight on the heels as the bar descends down the thigh. The ability to take up the slack in the hamstrings by having good intent with weight through the midfoot at the start of the top of the movement is also lost with this strategy.

Starting with the weight through the midfoot and then travelling back towards the heel while maintaining some pressure through the midfoot will create a movement that is genuinely challenging the athlete's base of support and will cause them to react subconsciously in order to maintain balance.

As the athlete descends with the barbell, the knees should straighten slightly to fully overcome hamstring slack while the humerus should externally rotate in order to take up the slack in the transverse plane of the latissimus dorsi by externally rotating the humerus.

By taking up all the slack, this allows the athlete to transmit forces well through the thoracolumbar fascia, through the hands, and through the thoracolumbar fascia into the hamstrings and glutes.

As the athlete ascends and returns to the start position, I would ideally like to see the weight distribution travel forwards towards midfoot and forefoot as the hips genuinely travel forward. A lack of intent through midfoot and forefoot will usually result in excessive lumbar extension rather than true hip extension and we lose the ability to stimulate the distal hamstrings and proximal glutes in the lift.

Also ensuring the weight travels forward will again force the athlete to manage their base of suppose as the weight shifts forwards with hip extension.

Squat

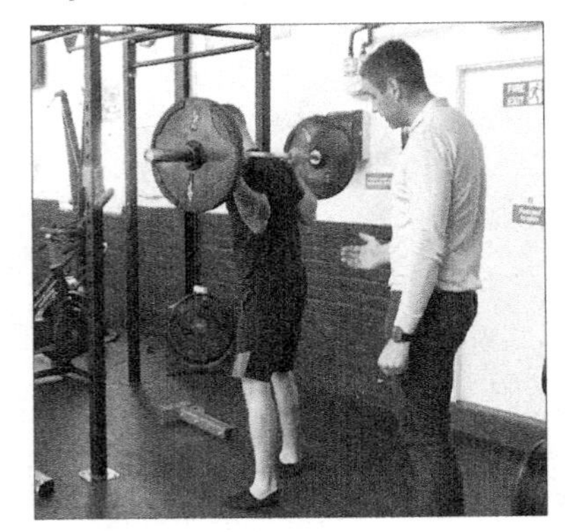

The weight needs to start in the midfoot before the descent in the squat. As the body descends, weight should travel towards the heels while maintaining some pressure in the foot through the midfoot and forefoot.

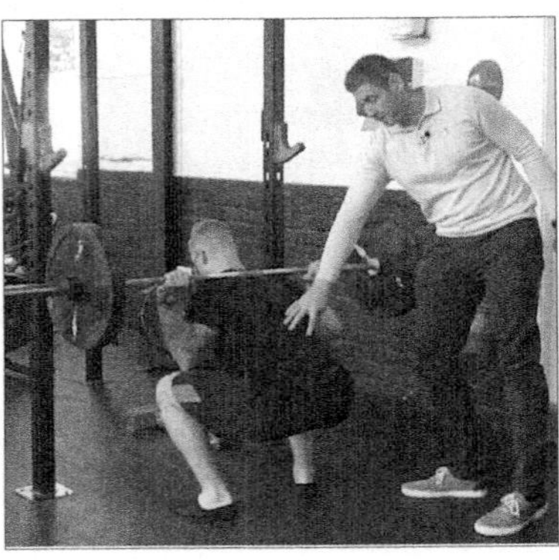

At the bottom of the squat, the intent is initially to push through the heels and midfoot and as the bar ascends and the hips travel upwards and forwards, the intent must then come towards the midfoot and forefoot at the end of the movement with a clear forward movement of the hips over the foot. An inefficient strategy often seen in the intent is through the heels throughout the ascent. This will then cause the knees to snap back with an excessive extension of the lower back instead of through hip extension movement.

The biggest mistake I see with the squat movement is the athlete starting with the weight distribution already on the heels. If the athlete starts with the weight distribution on the heels, as they go back in hip flexion, the weight is already there and the distribution has ultimately nowhere else to go. In my experience, this usually results in the athlete excessively leaning forward at the trunk.

As the athlete starts the movement, the weight distribution should be around the midfoot and as they are descending to the squat, it should go towards the heels while still maintaining some amount of pressure through the midfoot to forefoot. If I was forced to put a percentage on it, I would say at the bottom of the squat I would like 60% of the force through the heels and 40% through the midfoot to forefoot. As we ascend into hip extension, I would like to see this percentage reversed.

Please note this is just my opinion on what feels right after studying the muscle architecture, gait and Olympic lifting foot pressures. I would love to see some formal studies being performed on this with the difference in muscle activation and foot pressure strategies as I think it is very important to movement variability.

Anyway, as the athlete comes out of the squat, the weight distribution should go from the heels towards the forefoot, from my observations. This would neurologically make sense in my mind as this is the same foot pressure distribution that has to happen during the gait cycle and also in Olympic lifting.

Once you get your athletes to restore full weight distribution through the foot, you will see that the gluteus activation takes care of itself and there is no need to 'squeeze the glutes' at the top of the lift. The majority of the pressure is through the forefoot which ultimately helps take up slack in the system and increases the tone around the proximal gluteus maximus without having to squeeze the glutes and extend the lumbar spine which so many athletes appear to be doing these days.

Press-ups

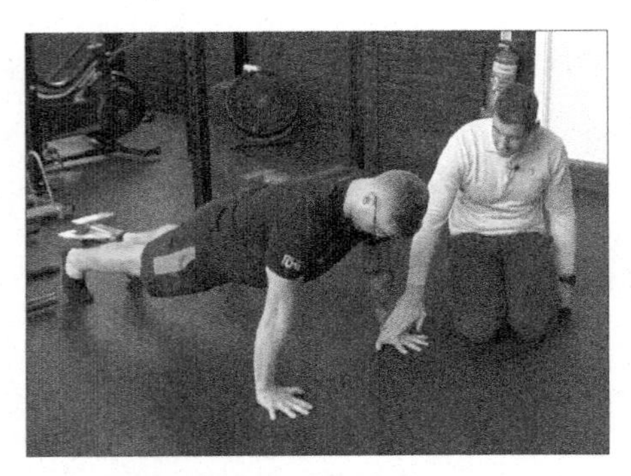

At the start of the press-up position, the weight should be through the mid-hand. As the athlete descends, the weight should then travel to the heel and outside the hand while inhaling slowly to control the elevation of the ribcage and to avoid overarching the lower back.

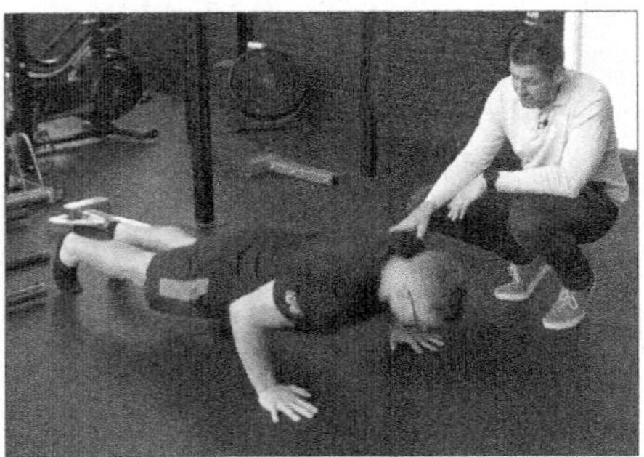

Similar to the squat, at the bottom of the movement, the intent is initially through the heel of the hand and then as the body ascends, the weight must shift towards the mid-hand and fingers to maximise the contribution of the distal triceps and forearm flexors which are often underutilised in these movements. This will help promote greater movement variability and variance of movement.

The biggest mistake I see with press-ups is the athlete holding their breath and not allowing the ribcage to mobilise. As the athlete descends in the press, we can facilitate the ribcage into extension with a nice controlled inhale which will control the ribcage via the diaphragm. This would straight away take care of excessive arching of the back and/or neck as the diaphragm contracting would help facilitate the elevation of the ribcage.

Another issue with press-ups is not allowing the weight to distribute through the full hand. Usually the weight is kept on the heel of the hand which is ultimately then going to stimulate only certain portions of the muscles as they transmit force through the floor via the hand through the torso. As the athlete pushes back to the start position, there should be good intent through the mid-hand and fingers also to help distribute forces well to the triceps and posterior deltoid while also using the wrist flexors which are very important for contact sports and are often under-trained due to poor hand weight distribution.

Rowing/pulling movements

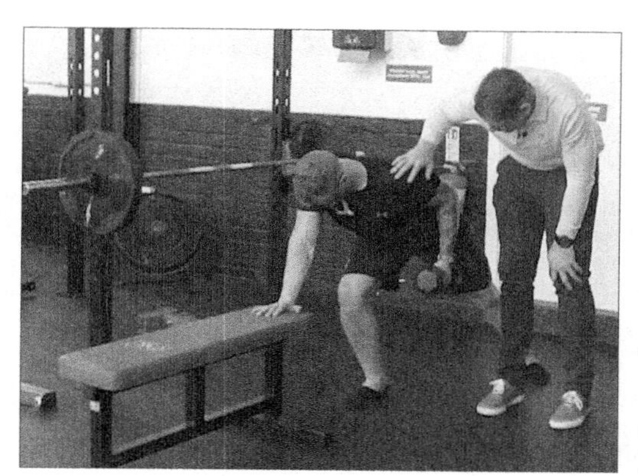

Ensure that the stance hand has a co-contraction at the elbow joint and the weight is distributed through the heel, mid-hand and fingers evenly to promote stability through the distal elbow muscles and forearm flexors also. Initiate the row with intent from the fingertips to again promote forearm flexors and pull towards the hip.

One of the biggest mistakes I see on a daily basis with rowing or pulling type movements is pulling the elbow too high towards the mid ribcage and not towards the hip. This usually results in the upper trapezius shrugging upwards rather than true scapula retraction.

If we can get the athlete to pull towards the hip, then usually we get a much nicer retraction with the scapula posterior tilting rather than being downwardly rotated.

I also like the intent of the pull to happen from the fingertips to ensure we stimulate the wrist flexors during the movement and allow them to contribute their fair share of work to the movement.

The opposite hand also must ensure that it takes up slack while performing a row in order to keep the athlete safe to distribute the external loads through the body, down through to the ground via the feet and also down to the bend or support with this hand. An athlete that's not actively taking up the slack here may leave themselves vulnerable to transmitting forces in various directions through the thoracolumbar fascia from my experience and not directing these forces well through the body which ultimately results in them being absorbed excessively in a certain area.

Overhead pressing

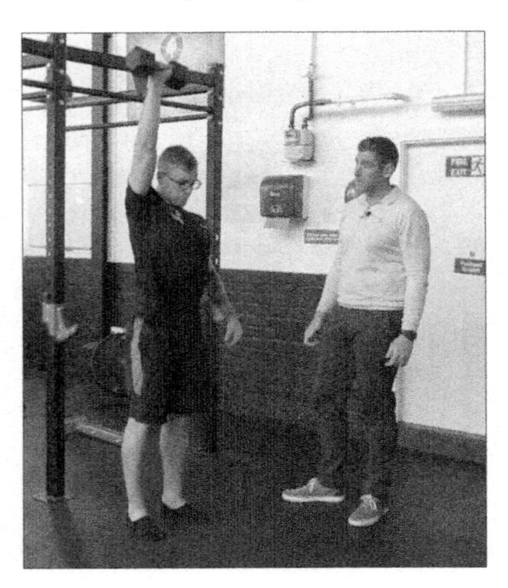

Ensure that the tongue is placed on the roof of the mouth to help the deep neck flexors' length tension relationship be more advantageous to offering the neck stability through the movement which will then allow the levator scapulae to lengthen as the scapula protracts and upwardly rotates throughout the press.

One of the biggest mistakes that is common with overhead pressing is an incorrect tongue position, believe it or not. The athlete's tongue should rest on the roof of the mouth just behind the teeth which will ultimately take up the slack in the deep neck flexor tissues. An inability to take up the slack in the deep neck flexors may be problematic for the athlete and they will search for other ways to overcome muscle slack such as excessive neck extension.

From my experience dealing with injuries that were triggered from overhead pressing, the levator scapulae tries its best to offer stability to the cervical spine in some form of extension or side flexion of the neck. The problem arises when the athlete wants to push a weight overhead and the scapulae needs to upwardly rotate and protract which would require it to lengthen.

The levator scapulae now has a difficult decision. It needs to allow tissues to lengthen distally when the scapula needs to move with the arm overhead while also needing to work to provide stability at the cervical spine.

From my experience, I believe the levator scapulae and even serratus posterior tissues may go into some form of protective tone when the system perceives a threat and ultimately results in a cervical disc-like presentation of an athlete after lifting overhead.

If you can rectify all the strategies mentioned above and you can get the athlete to lift well with plenty of movement variability, then this can be a massive piece of the puzzle solved in ensuring that your injury prevention system is effective. If you address every other section, but the athlete continues to lift poorly in the gym, then your Injury Prevention Machine will always be placing excessive strain on certain parts.

Summary of key points

The coaching cue of push through the heels when lifting is causing more harm than good from my experience. The majority of athletes are starting the lift with all the weight on their heels which results in a lack of weight distribution through the foot. This affects the ability of the distal hamstrings and proximal gastrocnemius to co-contract at the knee efficiently and to allow the hip joint to do genuine work. The quadriceps tend to do excessive work and the knees snap back, with the lower back then having to hyper extend at the top of the lift and the athlete consciously squeezing the glutes. Starting with the weight through the midfoot and then the weight travelling towards the heels as the hip goes into flexion, and the weight distribution going towards the midfoot as the hip extends, allows an opportunity for the athlete to manage perturbatory loads subconsciously and to manage their base of support. This will also utilise the distal hamstrings and proximal gastrocnemius and promote a more efficient co-contraction at the knee joint, delaying knee extension so the hip joint can do more work.

CHAPTER 9

The force absorption production micro system

A big focus in the injury prevention system specifically implemented in the pre-training movement prep and warm-up prior to field is the force absorption micro system.

The ability of an athlete to decelerate their body weight and put their foot in an optimal position to produce force into the ground is critical to athletic success and is often overlooked, in my experience.

The majority of athletes that have experienced lower limb symptoms and tendon problems usually tend to lack awareness of the midfoot intent during the deceleration. The athlete will usually use a forefoot and toe strategy to decelerate and find their centre of mass too far forward when reproducing force. The heel may also lift off the floor early which can cause the soleus and quadriceps to work excessively.

The ability to decelerate and find the midfoot is advantageous and attractive to us as therapists and performance coaches as pushing through midfoot to forefoot will allow better plantar flexion forces and manage horizontal ground reaction forces better.

The ability of the distal hamstrings and gastrocnemius to engage and co-contract at the knee joint with the quadriceps will protect the knee joint, and the ACL in particular, with midfoot intent.

The real advantage of midfoot intent is that it gives us movement options for the next step.

If the athlete decelerates excessively with the forefoot/toes, it is very difficult to then have to pivot and turn back towards the direction they came as the centre of mass travels forward of the base of support and it is more difficult to produce force horizontally into the ground to push the body back in the opposite direction.

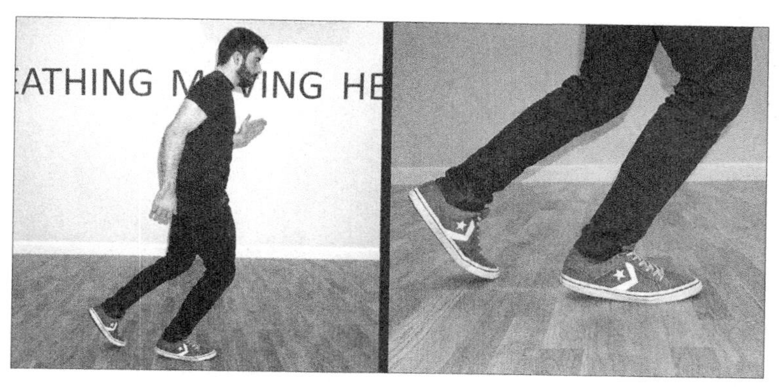

Notice the athlete's centre of gravity is slightly forward and almost falling forward which is suboptimal if he needs to suddenly pivot and turn in reaction to an opponent.

If the athlete decelerates excessively through the heel and then has to reaccelerate forwards or cut forwards and sideways, the body mass is slightly behind the base of support and not in the optimal position to produce force horizontally into the floor to move forwards.

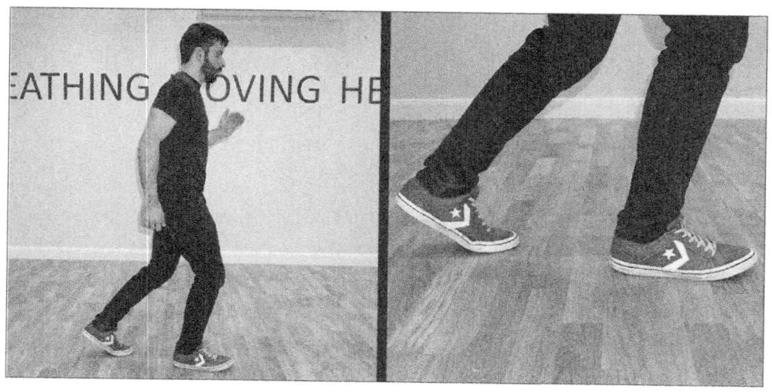

Notice the athlete's centre of gravity is slightly behind him which makes him vulnerable if he was to go into contact with an opponent.

The ability to find the midfoot/forefoot before reproducing force into the floor is attractive as it gives us balance as the centre of mass is over the base of support and the athlete now has options to apply force horizontally with the intention of going forwards, backwards, sideways and twisting while utilising the majority of lower limb muscles as needed.

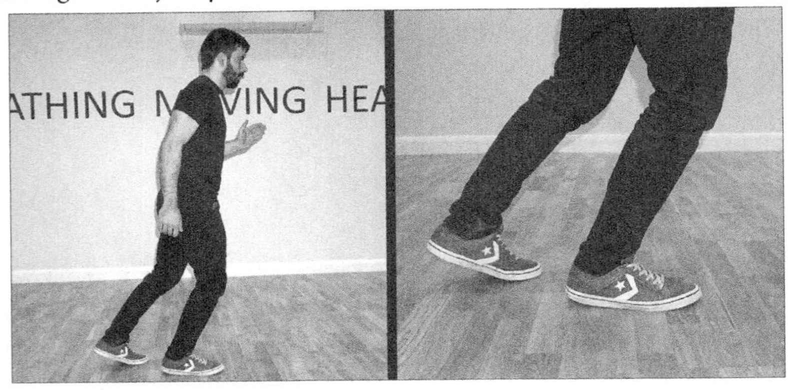

Notice the athlete's centre of gravity is now between his base of support and is more balanced to give and take contact, react to an opponent and move forward or back and also be able to cut and side step. In other words the athlete has the ability to put force into the floor and move in numerous directions for his next step.

In other words we have movement options and can manage the ground reaction forces and possible external loads through the whole limb without overloading certain tissues or tendons to adjust for poor force absorption capabilities.

I hope you can now also see the importance of ensuring the midfoot is utilised and stimulated in the gym as discussed in the previous chapter to help the athlete move well on the field.

The ability to accelerate and decelerate to a complete stop over 10 metres at maximal effort and distributing the load through the midfoot while stopping in a balanced position can be very challenging for even world-class athletes. Going straight into these drills in pre-season can be very risky as the inability to do these drills well can often lead to excessive load going through the patella tendon or sometimes the Achilles tendon. From my experience, old adductor and groin issues can be aggravated. This is why in the force absorption production micro system, it is important that we work towards this end goal in a graded exposure manner in order to minimise 'perceived threats' from the nervous system.

As mentioned already, it will usually take me anywhere between 6 to 12 weeks before we work up to these progressions in the movement prep.

For a more in-depth look at my progressions to get the athlete to be able to decelerate at high speeds and high loads please see my other book *The 'Go To' Physio* as I cover each progression in more detail there.

But in a nutshell here is how the graded exposure focused on the force absorption production would look from pre-season into in-season:

Weeks 1–2: Holding lunge positions with good co-contraction of the knee joint and body weight travelling over midfoot and sticking in a strong athletic position with movement options in all three planes of motion. This movement will be done with a sagittal, frontal and transverse plane bias of each direction.

Weeks 3–4: Leaping from one leg to the other and landing in a good midfoot position with good co-contraction of the knee joint and body weight travelling over midfoot and sticking in a strong athletic position with movement options in all three planes of motion. This movement will be done with a sagittal, frontal and transverse plane bias of each direction.

Weeks 5–8: Hop and stick on one leg and landing on same leg in a good midfoot position with good co-contraction of the knee joint and body weight travelling over midfoot; sticking in a strong athletic position with movement options in all three planes of motion. This movement will be done with a sagittal, frontal and transverse plane bias of each direction.

Weeks 9–10: Performing three to five hops on one leg and landing on same leg in a good midfoot position with good co-contraction of the knee joint and body weight travelling over midfoot; sticking in a strong athletic position with movement options in all three planes of motion. This movement will be done with a sagittal, frontal and transverse plane bias of each direction. The intensity may increase from 50% maximal effort to upwards of 100% after each set.

Weeks 11–12 onwards: Jog five steps and stick landing on same leg in a good midfoot position with good co-contraction of the knee joint and body weight travelling over midfoot and sticking in a strong athletic position with movement options in all three planes of motion. This movement will be done with a sagittal, frontal and transverse plane bias of each direction. The intensity may increase from 50% maximal effort to upwards of 100% after each set.

Each week we would still include the previous week's content but decrease the time spent on these and allocate two to three minutes more for the next progression.

After 12 weeks into the movement prep, sessions would contain high levels of hopping and deceleration progressions prior to the field sessions.

Please note, I cannot emphasise enough how important it is to earn the right to progress to each progression and not simply go to the 'sexy' high level with high load progressions. From my experience, this will usually cause flare-ups of old injuries.

During the process, any athletes who we feel need additional help with the deceleration progressions will work with the rehab conditioner pre-training as outlined in chapter 1 where they will spend additional time on the lower level progressions and earn the right to progress. During the movement prep sessions, they may be modified to the level of loading they would undertake if the current squad progressions were thought to be too high a level for them.

Time spent earning the right to progress to the higher level progressions in this micro system is time well spent on creating durable, resilient athletes.

It was only when new signings came to the club that I realised how far ahead my current athletes were and how much more energy-efficient they were in controlling their body weight and reproducing force into the ground.

To watch real-life examples of these deceleration progressions in the movement preparation sessions, please visit **www.injurypreventionbook.com/resources**

Summary of key points

The ability of the athlete to control their body weight when decelerating and put it in a good position over their base of support to reproduce force efficiently into the ground is a critical component to the injury prevention system. If the athlete decelerates excessively with the forefoot, it is very difficult to then have to pivot and turn back towards the direction they came, as the centre of mass travels forward of the base of support and it is more difficult to produce force horizontally into the ground to push the body back in the opposite direction. If the athlete decelerates excessively through the heel and then has to reaccelerate forwards or cut forwards and sideways, the body mass is slightly behind the base of support and not in the optimal position to produce force horizontally into the floor to move forwards. The ability to find the midfoot/forefoot before reproducing force into the floor is attractive as it gives us balance as the centre of mass is over the base of support and the athlete now has options to apply force horizontally with the intention of going forwards, backwards, sideways or twisting while utilising the majority of lower limb muscles as needed. The athlete needs to earn the right to progress through the structured deceleration progressions in order to minimise 'perceived threats' or flare-ups from the nervous system.

CHAPTER 10

The soft tissue treatment strategies micro system

The role of the soft tissue massage therapist is vital in order to ensure that your injury prevention system is robust. The ability to influence tone of tissues with our hands can be very advantageous but it can also be very disadvantageous. The 'Go To' Therapist understands that if we take away protective tone without addressing the reason for it, there may potentially be a greater reactive strategy once a stressor is placed upon that body part again or, even worse, the body will find another body part or area to transfer forces which may eventually result in protective tone in this area.

One of the rules in my last three years with the Huddersfield Giants was that no player was allowed to get his hamstring and low back massaged. The reason behind this was simple. We needed to stop treating the tissues that were giving the symptoms and rather ask ourselves why these tissues were becoming sensitised in the first place, giving these sensations of tightness.

It was very easy to remove the need to get these tissues massaged and appease the athlete by addressing other areas of the body that were not moving as efficiently as we would like.

The 'Go To' Therapist appreciates the reaction that the loss of the ability of the diaphragm to lengthen will result ultimately in the tissues of the athlete's posterior chain hamstrings to potentially lengthen as a result of a now secondary elevated ribcage position.

Think going to touch your toes while keeping your chest proud (or your ribcage elevated). You will feel tension in your hamstrings very quickly, similar to an RDL movement. Now repeat but completely relax your neck and slouch before touching your toes while actively reaching with your fingertips.

This will help drive the ribcage to be depressed and you should feel you are a lot closer to the floor before you notice your hamstring tissues.

This certainly made sense in my mind that if the fascial and skin receptors were simply becoming sensitised and giving this experience of tightness due to being stimulated, is lengthening or stimulating them further the real solution?

Massaging those tissues in theory would just further sensitise them. And, although the athlete may get a reflexive change initially, usually, from my experience, the symptoms return quickly.

The lower back and, in particular, the erector spinae tone is one area that I'm very slow to go about influencing with hands-on treatment. The 'Go To' Therapist has been taught to ask some serious questions about the tone of this tissue. 'Why is the tone of these tissues so high and why has the system perceived this to be of value in order to keep this person ultimately safe? Therefore, is 'loosening' and taking away this tone really a good thing for this person at this moment in time passively?'

From my experience, as this is such an important part of the body, which has to absorb and deal with lots of movement errors within the rest of the body, it may not be the best idea to take the tone out of these tissues if we have not found the reason for them absorbing errors in the first place.

Or, put more simply, loosening these tissues short-term without finding the areas of the body not doing their own job may cause a further 'perceived threat' once the load is increased again in the real world.

On one occasion in 2012, I remember it was the day before the semi-final of the play-offs. A senior player got on the massage bed and asked for their lower back tissues to be massaged quickly as their lower back was feeling tight. Against our policy, the soft tissue therapist did it anyway without informing me or the assistant physiotherapist as it was a senior player and they wanted to appease them. Low and behold, ten minutes into the team run, the player's right gluteal muscle went into extreme spasm and the player had to withdraw from the training session.

My hypothesis on this occasion was that we took away the player's protective strategy in the form of high tone around the lower back so the nervous system self-organised and recruited stability through the gluteus medius and deep rotator tissues in terms of protective tension.

Now, on this occasion, I was able to trace back the true stressor to the player and give him back the ability to put forces in these directions so the body did not feel the need to apply this protective tone. We were able to reassure the system that it was safe, restore the tone of the gluteus medius and the player was able to successfully take part in the semi-final the following night. However, it took a little bit of work for me on the day of the training session and also some treatment before the game.

But we were lucky: on another occasion with a more extreme reaction from the nervous system, we might not have got the player through the game.

This is a clear example to me of taking away protective tone of the body without appreciating the consequences of our actions. Therefore, a soft tissue therapist needs to be extremely careful and to be aware that when we take away protective tone in the short term, there may be consequences within the system to self-organise as a result of this tone being altered. Obviously I appreciate this is very hard to prove scientifically but this is my observation from working in professional sporting environments day in, day out over the last ten years.

Therefore, the 'Go To' Therapist will always ask, 'Why is this tissue carrying this tone at the moment? Is there a reason?' As I teach on the ProSport Academy 'Go To' Therapist Mentorship, if we can find the true stressors, then very often the tone of this tissue will usually change also without having to directly treat this tissue.

There is ALWAYS a reason for high tone and it just takes a little bit of detective work, but if you start to ask better questions you will usually get better answers and you will find the true stressors to the patient or athlete's story.

Therefore, the soft tissue treatment plan for an athlete should always, in my opinion, have a reason for manually restoring tone on the tissue that makes sense and also be accompanied by some form of reassurance and graded exposure in terms of putting load through tissues, forcing the body to self-organise straight after taking away a protective tone. This can then ensure that we have earned the right to keep this tone long term without it increasing again at the first sign of increased stress on the system.

From experience, approaching the body in this way, I usually see long-lasting changes as opposed to just reflexive changes, where the athlete comes back in the following day with the same symptoms.

The pre-season screening will also give you valuable information about some areas of the body you might need to give some attention to in the forms of stimulating certain tissues in certain directions to help restore and reassure the tissues' ability to lengthen. The athlete's story is also a great place to look for some long-term protective tone that may be unknown to the athlete but causing other tissues to absorb forces in certain directions.

Following this approach, I have found our soft tissue strategies to be an integral part of our injury prevention system, provided it is not abused. We don't want to give an athlete the opinion that they need to rely on soft tissue strategies and they become over-reliant on passive therapies. By treating the athlete and then getting them to work actively throughout the session integrating or lengthening the diaphragm while having treatment can be very advantageous. It stops the athlete sitting there passively and expecting results without having to earn the right to keep them. Soft tissue treatment combined with the athlete taking an active role will stop this type of thinking or behaviour.

This type of approach is a big change for some medical departments and also for a lot of senior players. However, once the results come and the athlete can feel the difference in tone of the tissues and the long-lasting effects, they will usually accept this new approach with minimal fuss.

The above approach is a great way to set up your soft tissue system so that you only ever treat tissues if you have rationale for restoring the lengthening of these tissues. The 'Go To' Therapist asks if there is a genuine need to restore the lengthening or to desensitise the tissues. If so, then hands-on techniques may be appropriate. Far too often, it is too easy to have a tissue such as your glutes, your low back or your hamstrings with high tone and to simply massage the area.

In the old way of thinking, the therapist sends the athlete on their way having experienced reflexive changes but without realising or considering the consequences of taking away a protective tone of a tissue. We know too much about the reactions within and between muscles and noxious stimulus to continue with the old way of thinking.

In order to achieve best practice, we need to clinically reason every single thing that we do from the subjective assessment, right through to the return to play: this is ultimately my goal in the ProSport Academy 'Go To' Therapist Mentorship.

Looking at the soft tissues system in this approach was one of the best things that I've done and it also forced me to make some difficult decisions in finding the right people to manage my soft tissue therapy departments who were strong enough to not just appease the players but to deliver what the player actually needed rather than wanted.

Finding the right person is essential to achieving that ultimate continuum, so that what they do complements what you do and it also complements the athlete in helping them move while on the field and in the gym, recover well and get back into rest and digest. You can then start to appreciate the value of the whole team contributing bit by bit to the overall injury prevention system. You truly are only as strong as your weakest bolt in the Injury Prevention Machine.

Practically to help you implement this chapter in the real world, one of the major things we noticed from the pre-season screening was a lack of quadriceps lengthening ability and hip extension.

Therefore we ensured that the quadriceps soft tissue work was mandatory for every player at the end of every rub followed by an active assisted lengthening of these tissues with the therapist, to finish off the session. The players didn't like it at first as these tissues were sensitive; however they soon felt the benefits to their low backs and hamstrings and soon requested the quadriceps to be massaged of their own choice.

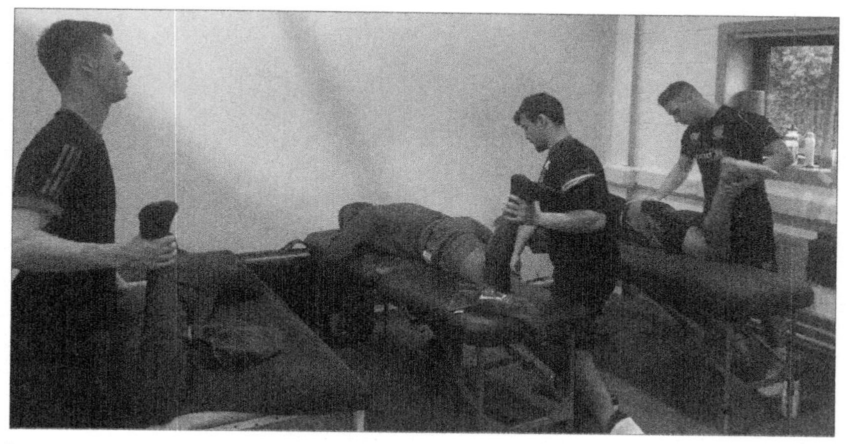

Players receiving active assisted lengthening of the quadriceps after every soft tissue session to help restore the lengthening ability of these tissues as identified by the pre-season and in-season screens. The quadriceps, and the vastus lateralis in particular, will absorb a lot of movement errors in my opinion for inefficient hamstrings and hips and therefore need to have the ability to absorb and produce force at all times. It is when these tissues' load tolerance is at capacity or has a reduced capacity, that we start to see symptoms appear elsewhere in the body as a reaction.

This in itself was a massive culture change and a small win from the usual request of massage to calves, hamstrings and low back; we soon started to see the transference to their movement capabilities in the gym and with their deceleration and movement prep work on a daily basis.

Summary of key points

The soft tissue therapist plays a key role in helping the athlete achieve athletic capabilities. The pre-season screening and daily markers data can be used to make clinically reasoned decisions about what the athlete needs rather than what they want. It takes a strong character to lead this role and implement a soft tissue system that prevents athletes becoming reliant on passive interventions. Understanding the impact of reflexive changes as a result of soft tissue therapy and the possible reactions is important for every soft tissue therapist to understand, especially when delivering interventions pre-training or game.

CHAPTER 11

Management of acute injuries micro system

Just as the soft tissue therapy team need to be efficient, it is also essential that the physiotherapist or sports therapist can manage acute and ongoing niggles fast and effectively. We will discuss specifically the acute management of injuries in regards ice and compression in the post-game management micro system but in this chapter I would like to discuss the ability to minimise motor adaptations to pain or noxious stimulus that may happen during the injury process.

In order to have a strong robust Injury Prevention Machine, the therapist must ensure the symptoms are addressed efficiently and don't cause further adaptations within the musculoskeletal system.

An ineffective management of acute injuries may present themselves in the form of other compensatory movement strategies that may have a significant contribution to a pain or unpleasant experience later down the line with further training or playing time lost, based on my experience of dealing with complex cases that have failed traditional approaches.

The ability of the therapist to have a clear understanding, a clear assessment strategy from the subjective assessment right through to return to play is absolutely essential in terms of preventing major injuries. While niggles and aches and pains are naturally occurring phenomenon, the ability to deal with these quickly and effectively can be the difference between an injury developing and having a very robust injury prevention system in place, in my opinion.

Just like the soft tissue therapist, the 'Go To' Therapist needs to ask the athlete appropriate questions to find the true stressor of the problem, make sense of the objective assessment, decrease that perceived threat, restore the ability of the tissues to shorten and lengthen and restore the ability to self-organise in particular directions when the tissues are under direct load. These things are of utmost importance in ensuring that the athlete does not lose movement variability. Losing movement options and variability of movement may potentially have more serious or sinister consequences in the form of injury or unpleasant sensations such as tightness.

In order to ask the appropriate questions and gain clarity on the contributing factors towards the pain experience and injury process, the physiotherapist or healthcare professional requires a refined system that understands the key fundamental principles that have been outlined in Chapter 2. Understanding the stressors and previous injuries that the athlete has had, not only this season, but last, and why now all of a sudden these tissues may have become sensitised can be a big clue to address the true stressors of the problem so that we can prevent further motor adaptations to noxious stimuli.

One thing that I used with the Huddersfield Giants towards the end of my tenure there was noting any bumps, dead legs or bruises that athletes picked up the day after a game. Now, although the athlete may not actively complain about these and would just see them as part of their day-to-day games and process of playing a contact sport, understanding how the body interacts with pain and stress may show us some potential issues further down the line. The 'Go To' Therapist could reason that these potentially innocuous bumps that may have almost gone unknown, could potentially manifest themselves and cause that athlete to alter the forced directions that they use now, in order to create a movement output around a particular joint or particular limb as a result of the original noxious stimulus during the acute stage. And we know from the literature that once the noxious stimulus is removed, a person may not necessarily return to their previous movement strategies, and motor adaptations may still be present.

Although we did not go into this in enough depth in order to carry out a clinical study, due to the demands and pressures of real world professional sport, we did find some interesting results. We found in some cases where athletes presented to us with 'aches and pains' or 'niggles', when we looked back at the records for the last two, three or four weeks of any bumps or bangs, we could on some occasions find a part of the body that had experienced direct trauma.

We would then assess those areas for the skin, the fascia, and the tissues to lengthen and shorten. We helped the athlete to reassure their system that it was safe to put through a force in this direction and then on a few occasions we were quickly able to successfully resolve the symptoms that the athlete had originally come in with, without lingering symptoms.

Now, although we need a lot more evidence and potential clinical trials to make any outrageous statements regarding this, it is an area that interests me at the moment; certainly if I was still actively in full-time professional sport, I would be looking into doing some form of structured research on it. I feel that understanding the motor adaptations and reactions between pain, trauma and the interaction with the musculoskeletal and nervous system will be of great value to the sports physio in the coming years.

The ability for the clinician to have a system in place where they can easily and effortlessly identify areas of the body to look at, restore and reassure, as well as lengthening and shortening the capacities of tissues and placing some load in these directions, can be of great value and is an essential component to having a robust injury prevention system.

My own thought process and 80/20 rule that I teach in my 'Go To' Therapist Mentorship is that 20% of my time and attention is focused on the site of the symptoms or pain experience while 80% of my time is spent on what I perceive to be the true stressor. This is usually an area of the body away from the site of pain which is not doing enough work and causes a 'perceived threat' that presents itself at the site of the symptoms.

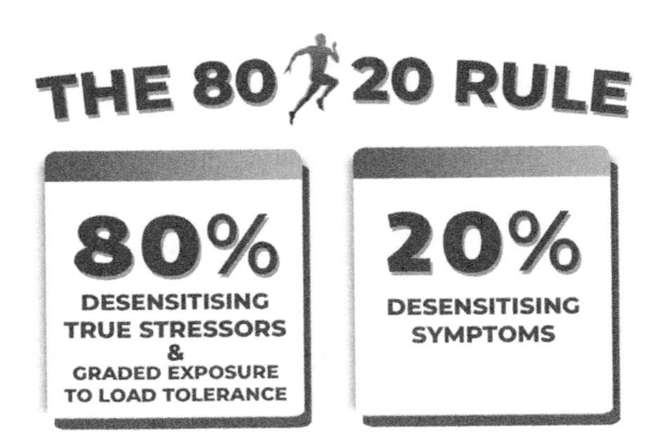

20% of the therapist's time should be spent on the pathology or desensitising the symptoms. 80% of the time should be spent desensitising the 'perceived threat' that caused the symptomatic area to overload in the first place along with a graded exposure of load reassurance.

Of course with a direct traumatic injury this may be slightly different but the ultimate aim in the acute stage is to maintain the nervous system's ability to load the limb or area in all directions and minimise motor adaptations to pain or the noxious stimulus.

The ability to stop excessive torque and force production in specific manners as a result of losing movement variability through that joint, or through those tissues originally injured, is of great value, in my opinion, in halting further adaptations that may present with some form of nociceptive stimulus that may contribute to the pain experience with some common injuries such as tendonitis, tendinosis etc that may present further down the line. Again I appreciate this is my own theory, but from my experience using this thought process has been consistently effective in minimising the amount of 'routine' non-traumatic injuries that usually present in rugby settings.

Once the main suspected stressors are addressed, it is imperative that the athlete's system is loaded in a progressive graded exposure manner to avoid further reactions or compensations.

When we appreciate the interactions that happen within the musculoskeletal system, we can see how important it is not to skip steps once the pain goes and the range of movement improves as there may still be underlying adaptations from the nervous system which may present themselves later on in contributing to other injuries. The advantage of having a robust, refined system is that the athlete has to go through a graded exposure programme throughout the week which may prove valuable in reducing further motor adaptations to noxious stimuli.

For example, if an athlete picked up an injury in a Sunday game and they had another game the following Sunday, the physio needs to have clarity on a graded yet intense return to play plan to decrease pain and restore the full range of movement objectively. Rather than putting the athlete straight back into training on a Wednesday and have them hobble through the session, the physio needs to load that athlete progressively over the course of two to three days and then put the athlete back into team training on a Friday so that they are able to take part fully on the Friday and Saturday sessions in order to make team selection for the Sunday.

While some may say this could upset coaches and that you are hanging onto players too long, if you can clinically reason exactly why you are following these steps then there should be no issue to the player or to the coach. If we skip steps and put an athlete straight back in once pain has resolved, from my experience the athlete will still show a decreased range of movement on, say, an ankle dorsiflexion range of movement pre-training marker consistently for two to three weeks. Although they are functioning well and they're getting through games, they will complain of an ache or a pain and some form of loss of range of motion will be seen throughout the next few weeks, or after games, and make your life more difficult in the coming weeks after they return to full training.

Compare this with our previous approach where taking that extra day, earning the right and progressively loading the athlete, making sure to tick all your boxes in terms of restoring length under load, stressing the axis of rotation that the injury occurred, observing the reactions and then putting the athlete back into training can have a massive effect further down the line.

Once there is pain, we have to respect that pain changes everything. If we can resolve that pain quickly and effectively, we can restore the motor output and load tolerance in this direction. We can also keep the range of movement at the original baseline without this ongoing niggly pain and loss of range of movement which may have consequences for that athlete's movement variability and capabilities down the line. If we can restore intent to produce force and access full range of motion, this can only be seen as a good thing versus getting through games okay but having that constant ache and pain and loss of range of movement to the present two, three, four weeks down the line.

The reality of the situation is two, three or four weeks down the line, you will have picked up on other athletes' injuries and you will naturally tend to forget about this athlete. They will go back into the cycle of the system and you may not see them again until further down the line where they may have picked up a traumatic or non-traumatic injury which may or may not have been related to this original ankle injury.

So, it is something to consider that you need to have a very focused and refined system where you understand what you need to achieve to help the athlete's nervous system move with 'thoughtless, fearless movement' and without negative motor adaptations, swelling and/or pain.

The athlete has to earn the right to go through your graded exposure programme step by step which will replicate the loads and speed of movements that they need to be able to tolerate once they go back into training.

Now, when you have a turnaround of six or seven days, your programme may need to be accelerated but the athlete still has to earn the right to progress to each level. You may go through three to four levels on one particular day. If the athlete responds well, and they don't show any signs of reactions then, from my own point of view, they can usually progress to the next level. Once they have the ability to do what we need them to do, then we can send them safely back into the training environment knowing that the athlete has earned a right to get there. Clinically, that athlete's pre-training marker tests will consistently be back to baseline and they will not complain of unpleasant sensations of aches or pains.

It is this subtle difference, in my opinion, that differentiates the good from the great sports therapist in the professional sports setting. Now, I would encourage you as a professional therapist to strive to justify and clinically reason each step of your return to play process rather than it just being a case of when the pain goes, send the player back again. We need some form of refined step-by-step progression that can assess the ability of the system to self-organise and to ensure that we are sending an athlete back in a durable and robust manner. Once that athlete achieves these progressions, this will fill the therapist with confidence in sending the player back into the training or game environment.

For a full in-depth view of each step of my return to play system that I use in both pro sport and private practice, please see my other book *The 'Go To' Physio*.

Summary of key points

From my experience, it is not the actual injury that can cause delays to return to play but rather the motor adaptations laid down by the nervous system as a result of pain or a noxious stimulus. The therapist needs to ensure that they can minimise and undo these adaptations using a common sense graded exposure programme that exposes the athlete to the loads and speed of movements that they will need to tolerate when returning to their training environment. Simply returning an athlete to the training environment once pain has gone is not an efficient strategy as motor adaptations may still be present under higher loads and higher speeds of movement. Having a structured common sense step-by-step system is therefore critical to reassure the athlete's nervous system it is safe to tolerate load in the specific directions where there is a perceived threat.

CHAPTER 12

The pre-game micro system

On game day, your role changes slightly from during the week. During the week, the 'Go To' Therapist needs to be a very authoritative figure in terms of running pre-training markers, getting your movement prep sessions done, etc. and ensuring that the athletes respect what they need to do, respect your routines and do them to the best of their ability.

On game day, I tend to change my authoritative role a bit and I take a step back and let athletes prepare to the best of their ability to perform. Although it could be argued you should do pre-training markers on game day, personally, I decided not to do these provided that they were OK the day before the game and no incidents happened in the team or on the training session on that day.

In this scenario, if there was a player that had maybe rolled an ankle or hurt themselves, we might potentially do the pre-training markers with that particular player. But as a squad overall, I try to focus before the game on making the athletes feel as good as possible so that they can do their thing without having them worry about doing pre-training markers; rather than interfere with their pre-game routine, I just let them do what they need to do to perform to the best of their ability. On the other hand, if you choose to do pre-game markers in the dressing room on game day, I can completely respect and understand that too.

Ironically, the interesting thing that happened with the Giants was that when we brought in all the movement prep movements, naturally a few players whinged and moaned about doing them. But once they experienced how good they felt when going on field and how much quicker they could start and get into sessions, they bought into doing them. And it was these same players that you would see doing your movement prep movements pre-game on their own without being asked to do so.

So, my role on game day would be to step back into the shadows. I would strap ankles and I would let the player pretty much get any strapping that he needed to get through game day, whereas during the week I would ban strapping ankles unless there was an acute injury. I personally did not want the players to be relying on strapping, but on game day if they felt the need for strapping in their 'head', then usually the player would be allowed it. As the weeks went on and they were banned from strapping ankles for training, very often a lot of players dropped the ritual of getting their ankle strapped for games, which was encouraging from my point of view, and showed they believed in the resilience of their own bodies.

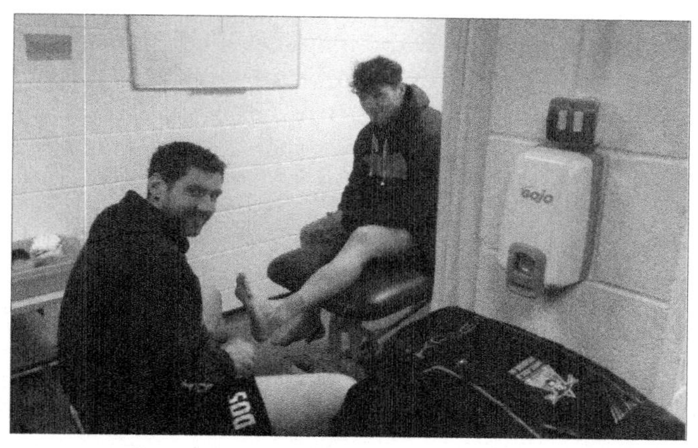

Players were not allowed to get their ankles strapped for training during the week unless there was an acute issue, but on game day they were allowed to do what they needed to do to feel right going into the game. As the weeks progressed, a lot of players weaned themselves off feeling the need to strap their ankles.

In terms of pre-game routine, one thing that we did was to do a five-minute movement prep before the players went out onto the field to do the warm-up with strength and conditioning coaches.

Now, this five-minute pre-game routine served twofold:

1. **It ensured that we prepared the athlete through four or five key movements in order to help them in that graded exposure manner to go to the field.**

2 **But it also helped them to tune in collectively as a team and served as a trigger to prepare them mentally and physically for what was to come. In this five-minute session, we ultimately aimed for ultimate coherence between the team. So every rep was done together. Every muscle/tissue lengthened and loaded was done on the same side and at the same time. Every repetition was done as a team. To encourage the team during this pre-game routine, I would use words that complemented the key messages that the head coach delivered prior to this movement prep.**

We would work a lot behind the scenes with the psychologist in terms of the words we use in order to bring the players into the present moment at any available opportunity when performing every single rep. What we wanted were the players to be in the 'here and now' while performing the movements. We did not want the players' minds to wander too far ahead, too far behind.

As advised by the psychologist, we wanted them in the present moment. This routine served us well over the three years with the Huddersfield Giants, not only helping us improve their movement prep, but also their readiness to play, go into game mode and deliver.

We saw this pre-game movement prep as another opportunity to expose the players to loads placed upon their bodies in a nice graded exposure before experiencing the more supra maximal loads that they would undertake in the actual games.

By exposing the nervous system to these loads, the hope was that the survival 'reactions' and instinct from the subconscious mind to these supra maximal loads would not be excessively over exaggerated or directly influence the movement variability and indeed the movement capabilities of the athlete.

One thing to note is that due to space restrictions of the dressing room, in this pre-game prep we focused predominantly on mobility and low level deceleration. The higher level deceleration work was performed as part of the warm-up as taken by the strength and conditioning coach.

At half-time, the players were checked and at full-time, we would usually check and manage the players as discussed in the next chapter.

Summary of key points

On game day, the main focus is on making the players feel confident and helping them become present in the 'here and now'. Pre-game markers are not done unless there is an ongoing issue or one occurs on the previous day. The pre-game movement prep focuses predominantly on mobility and lower level deceleration progressions prior to the players going out for warm-up while the higher level deceleration progressions are carried out on the field as part of the main warm-up with the strength and conditioning coach. The language used on game day is all positive and attention is placed on getting the players' minds on the 'here and now'.

CHAPTER 13

The post-game management of injuries micro system

From my own clinical experience, the way in which we manage an injury straight after a game is crucial in getting an athlete playing the following week. For instance, if a player reports that they rolled their ankle in the game, I would always be overcautious rather than under cautious after a game. Now, whether that means putting the athlete in an aircast boot, or strapping and compression over the ankle joint straight after the game until I saw how his/her nervous system reacted overnight, so be it.

If I had any suspicion of a syndesmosis type mechanism then I would always 'boot' the athlete straight after the game. Every athlete is different and every athlete responds differently, especially overnight to injuries. Therefore I would rather err on the side of caution for the first 12–24 hours.

I would rather have that player in the 'boot' because, from my experience, trying to make up days later on in the week is very, very hard if the initial 24 hours after the injury were not managed really well. I've seen some really bad syndesmosis injuries take onwards of up to 12 weeks to heal due to, in my opinion, the mismanagement straight after a game of that particular injury.

So, it's essential that you overreact rather than under-react to injuries straight after because we don't know for sure the reaction that the nervous system is going to produce in terms of swelling, in terms of pain once that athlete has got home, and throughout the night. Whereas if we have some form of compression to the area, that will usually limit the amount of swelling to some extent.

Offloading the injured site short-term (maximum 12 hours) may also potentially limit the reactions of the nervous system to the now sensitised tissues in the form of swelling. If we can limit the swelling, then we've got a greater chance of increasing the range of movement, restoring the ability of the tissues to shorten or lengthen and produce forces in any given direction earlier, and hence reduce the motor adaptations in the process. Whereas, usually if the swelling has been present and there is an 'overreaction' from the nervous system for a potential ankle sprain, then the additional swelling could potentially cost us a day or two in restoring range of motion and progressing the athlete to do what we need them to do in order to earn the right to get back into the training environment.

The inability to manage the athlete acutely after a game could potentially cost us two or three days in getting them to the next level on the return to play progression ladder in order for us to be confident that that athlete is safe first and foremost to progress. Reducing the reactions from the nervous system in the first few days will buy us time to work on restoring and reassuring the nervous system to load these tissues again with 'thoughtless, fearless movement'.

From experience, the ability to compress an injury is of the utmost value straight after a game, if possible. This is even true for traditional 'muscle' symptoms where the athlete may feel a tightening or an ache – it's important to get some form of compression there so that we can in theory stop any excessive overreaction of swelling if there was to be a chemical reaction.

Obviously, we need to appreciate that swelling is useful to the natural healing process but, in reality, very often the nervous system tends to overreact to even the smallest of injuries. Usually then, it's a case of waiting for the swelling to leave as opposed to the actual injury itself being a problem. The 'Go To' Therapist has got into the habit of having a good acute injury care after a game and does the basics extraordinarily. Getting into the practice of doing everything we can to prevent excessive swelling can have a massive effect on your ability to turn around players really quickly versus spending two, three days just working on the inflammation, from my own clinical experience.

In addition, good practice from the 'Go To' sports therapist will be to go around the dressing room at half-time to quickly check that each player is

OK. Quickly checking each player individually before the coach speaks to them is a good habit to get into and then also again straight after the game so you don't miss anything.

This may seem like something small but getting a check on each player where you physically make contact with the player and ask them, 'Are you OK? Is there any problem?' is of great value in identifying any potential issues that an athlete might not even think to tell you about after the game but might come in the following day with a swollen limb etc. If a player mentions anything of potential significance I would usually ask the player to come into the physio room before the shower, have a quick look and if we felt then that there was any risk of swelling happening overnight or any risk of potential issues then we would be overcautious rather than under cautious straight after a game. This, in practice led to no surprises the following day. By minimising the amount of surprises, we then have a fair idea of where we were at in terms of prognosis in giving the coach a quick injury report after the game and also the following day in regards who may not be available for the game the following week.

This kind of practice allows us to be confident in our decision-making in terms of predicting when this player will return to training as well as if they will be available for selection in the coming weeks. It can also help us give a better prognosis on when a player will be returning to training in the coming weeks if we have minimised swelling early on and are now working on the essential progressions.

I would recommend not committing to a prognosis or timescale until the next day and you can see how the nervous system has reacted overnight as sometimes injuries that seem minor can present the following day looking more serious; and so this saves the embarrassment of getting incorrect timescales. I would usually say 'we will need to see how it settles overnight and will have a better idea in the morning'. This buys you time and allows you to make a more informed decision rather than having to give one straight away. Coaches can be very emotional after games from my experience and can say all sorts of strange things to the press so it's best to keep it simple and positive.

Restoring the ability to access rest and digest post-game and training

Although we are in the post-game recovery micro system, all of the below information is also very much applicable to post-training recovery on a daily basis.

One of the big problems that I see in pre-season training and in games is the athlete's reliance on their sympathetic nervous system. While we will naturally gear towards our sympathetic nervous system through a day, the stresses and loads, both mentally and physically being placed upon professional athletes have never been greater.

The problem ultimately lies in the athlete's inability to access their parasympathetic nervous system frequently enough and especially once they have finished training or a game. This can lead players to struggle to sleep after games and the quality of sleep will be poor usually.

If we look at the setup of the day for an athlete, they spend the majority of their day in fight or flight. Some athletes continue to be stimulated even when on the massage bed with such devices as phones in their hands.

Now, one of the rules that I always had in place in my treatment room was that mobile phones were banned on the massage or physiotherapy beds. Besides the fact that it is just outright rude looking at your phone while you're getting a massage or treatment, the ability of the therapist to help your system get to a point of rest and digest will actually be influenced potentially by the stimulation received from phones.

We need to take any opportunity we have to help an athlete achieve a state of 'rest and digest' and an opportunity to get out of fight or flight, especially at the end of the day.

In order to recover efficiently after a game or training we must ask the question 'What truly is recovery for an athlete?'

Recovery, in my opinion is the ability to get back to a previous baseline or ultimately homeostasis, if that is even possible. For a lot of athletes, they are living predominantly in 'sympathetic dominance' and this becomes a habit. An ability to recover for them would simply be an ability to access the parasympathetic dominance at certain parts of the day.

When is it important to be able to recover to 'parasympathetic dominance'? Well, once the athlete has finished training certainly springs to mind but also it would be extremely important that the athlete is in 'parasympathetic dominance' before they go to sleep and when asleep so they can genuinely recharge, recover and be ready to go again. Recent studies are showing the link between sleep and injury prevention.

The work I do with heart rate variability and persistent pain patients clearly shows (using heart rate variability monitors) that the length of sleep is not the important thing but the *quality* of sleep. The ability to sleep in 'rest and digest' is very important for the body to recover and replenish. Some patients I've tracked can be getting eight plus hours of sleep but as little as one hour of that could be in the parasympathetic state which is needed for regeneration and recovery.

Usually, recovery sessions such as static stretching and swimming, etc. may to a point help the athlete get towards rest and digest but does it really address our physiology in any meaningful way?

The 'Go To' Therapist understands that a common reaction to stress is for the diaphragm and pelvic floor to carry high tone. A far more effective strategy is to give the athlete some form of exercise that's going to help them restore the ability to lengthen and shorten the diaphragm and also stimulate the vagus nerve.

One such exercise is humming. Yes, humming! Simply by putting your tongue on the roof of your mouth, lips together, breathing in through your nose and then humming for as long as you can is a great way to lengthen the diaphragm, stimulate the vagus nerve and prolong the period of time that the athlete spends in exhalation.

Inhalation is the system in a state of 'sympathetic dominance' while exhalation is a state of 'parasympathetic' dominance, therefore spending more time in the exhalation state is a great thing to do. When the athlete spends more time in exhalation, we are going to desensitise the ability of the diaphragm to lengthen again. We're going to spend more time with the heart rate decreased and we're going to spend more time in the parasympathetic side of our autonomic nervous system.

Humming essentially serves a few purposes: it increases the lengthening ability of the diaphragm, it prolongs the exhalation period subconsciously, it increases the time we spend in the parasympathetic side of the autonomic nervous system, it increases the time that our heart rate and blood pressure are decreased and it also increases the time for the oxygen to pump around the body and deliver to the cells. The 'Go To' Sports Therapist understands that this is a great activity to help an athlete truly recover and access a state of 'rest and digest'.

Therefore, spending one-on-one time with an athlete, and showing them how to perform an exercise like humming can provide invaluable rewards in the form of helping that athlete get back to 'rest and digest'.

The same problem arises in the evenings when the athlete goes home and their system has an inability to get to 'rest and digest'. Performing humming exercises, even silently without the noise can be a valuable exercise for an athlete before they go to sleep. Perform five minutes of silent humming with light, slow inhales between hums; once again this increases the lengthening at the diaphragm, decreases the sympathetic drive, increases the vagus tone and also helps the athlete to get into 'rest and digest' before going to sleep. It is an exercise that I use time and time again, despite what you may be thinking right now! I highly recommend it and it is very important, in my opinion, that we give athletes practical strategies that can take them from 'fight or flight' and back towards 'rest and digest' quickly and effectively.

Humming is also a great strategy that I've used in the past for players as they drive to training or when stopped at red lights. The advantage of this is that they are restoring the lengthening ability of the diaphragm and pelvic floor tissues so then once they get to training, you may see more satisfactory pre-training marker scores rather than the athlete having a stiff diaphragm and pelvic floor that's lost its ability to lengthen overnight due to the athlete being in 'sympathetic dominance' while asleep.

I would urge you to consider the use of some structured interventions and empower the athletes to take 5–10 minutes and help them with practical strategies to get into rest and digest.

Over the course of the three years with the Huddersfield Giants, we have used various strategies that have produced some great results in helping athletes restore their ability to get to 'rest and digest'.

Another form of accessing 'rest and digest' was taping athletes' mouths when they were getting soft tissue massage the day after a game. When we look at recovery strategies for an athlete, ultimately what we're trying to do is to take an athlete from 'fight or flight' back towards 'rest and digest'. Therefore, taping an athlete's mouth with paper tape would help them breathe through their nose for 30 minutes which would stimulate nitric oxide, which would then dilate the blood vessels and improve the oxygenation of the blood to the tissues. It also slows down our breathing rate and increases our breathing depth due to the pressure system exchange which then mobilises the diaphragm and pelvic floor and works towards improving our movement capabilities.

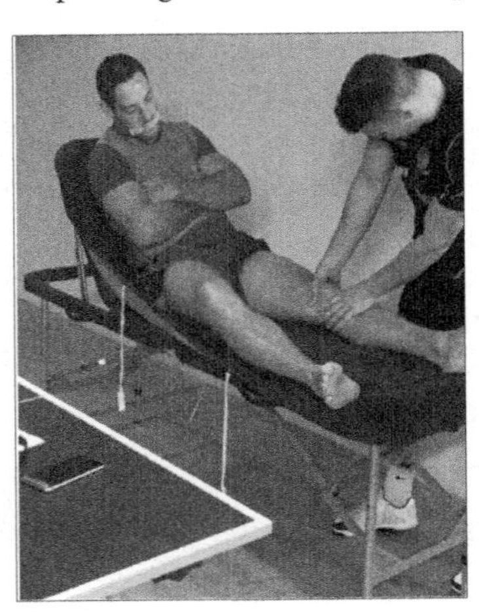

A player receiving a massage one-day post-game while having their mouth taped for 30 minutes to facilitate nasal breathing and to promote parasympathetic nervous system dominance.

Will you get some verbal abuse or some resistance from the athletes when asking them to put tape over their mouths? For sure. But the 'Go To' Therapist has authority over their athletes, they have the respect of their athletes and they have the belief from their athletes so, after all the huffing and puffing, they will trust you and feel the benefits of doing it.

(NB If an athlete has a deviated septum, or has a genuine reason for not being able to breathe through their noses, then you would not want to tape their mouth.)

Strategies such as humming and putting tape over athletes' mouths are great options to restore the athlete's ability to get back into 'rest and digest' and achieve true recovery. Their ability to sleep through the night will be improved as will their muscle soreness and ability to restore movement variability. In theory you should also be improving the ability of the diaphragm to lengthen and shorten and get back into 'rest and digest' after the demands of a pre-season training load or a daily training schedule for contact sports such as Rugby Union or Rugby League.

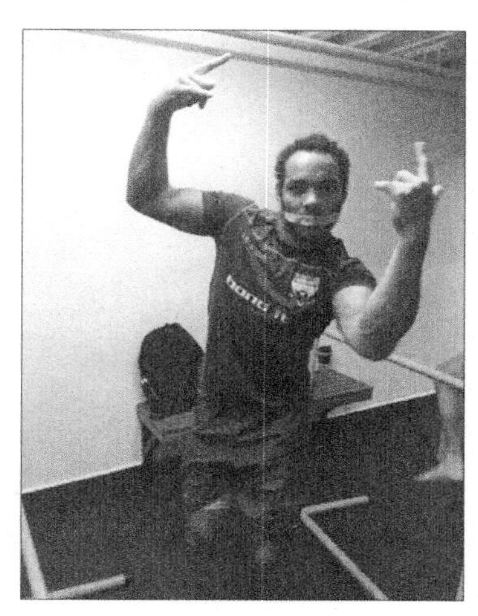

Players performing recovery session mobility exercises to restore range of motion while having their mouth taped to facilitate nasal breathing and to promote parasympathetic nervous system dominance.

The recovery session after games or the following day should again focus on restoring the lengthening ability of key peripheral tissues as well as desensitising the respiratory system using the strategies mentioned above.

Summary of key points

It is essential to overreact to injuries in the first 24 hours to minimise swelling and overreactions from the nervous system. Very often it will be excessive swelling that will delay progressing the athlete versus the injury itself. It is best to avoid committing to a prognosis until you have seen how the injury has reacted overnight as everyone's nervous system reacts differently to injury and/or pain. Helping the athlete to move away from sympathetic dominance and into parasympathetic dominance is critical for the athlete to truly recover and regenerate after training and while asleep. Practical strategies such as humming and taping the mouth to encourage nasal breathing are two strategies worth considering, integrated with the traditional stretching and mobility work, in order to desensitise the respiratory system.

CHAPTER 14

The communication micro system

This chapter is one you will not find covered in most undergraduate physiotherapy degrees yet it may be one of the most important concepts to understand to be a successful therapist in sport. The ability to maintain authority over players and staff is of the utmost importance to ensure you can actually implement the components of the Injury Prevention Machine outlined in previous chapters.

Professional sport in particular is a very high pressure environment that will have plenty of situations where you will have to make some quick decisions and deal with the consequences of those decisions. Now, as tends to happen in the real world, coaches and players can disagree with your decision-making and put pressure on you in order to attempt to return a player a little bit quicker than when they are ready, as discussed in the previous chapter.

With the best intentions in the world, you may go into a meeting or conversation and come out thinking 'Why did I just agree to let the player train/play this week?' How we get around this is maintaining authority at all times.

Authority in my own humble opinion is built upon many facets. First and foremost, having the utmost confidence in your own ability, knowledge and refined system allows you to portray this in your own physiology when communicating. Having a sound, logical and step-by-step progression allows you to clinically reason exactly where the athlete is in his/her return process and therefore justify exactly why it is safe or not safe for the athlete to return.

Another critical facet is communicating with the coach/player in his/her language. The majority of coaches and athletes will not care nor understand anatomical terminology and the meaning of your words. If we can talk in very easy to understand layman terms, then they too can logically understand the reasoning behind your decision-making process.

A final tip that I use when an athlete is not quite ready yet is to highlight the impact that the athlete not being right will have on the team. For instance, 'if the athlete pulls up ten minutes into the game, then your down a substitution already' or 'he will more than likely be a liability in the wrestle defensively this week if he were to play'. These are two examples where the coach can understand the implications of a player not being ready to return yet and how it affects the coach and team directly. Once the coach understands your reasoning process and the direct implications on the team, then I find they are quite straightforward to manage.

Establishing authority with players/athletes needs to be set from day one of working with a team or athlete. One way of establishing authority is to lay down the rules of how you run your medical department. When I went into the Huddersfield Giants at the end of 2012 for the 2013 season, it was still joked about three years later that one of the first things that I said to the players was, 'If you want my help, I will help you. If you don't want my help, and you are still in pain and you're not going to be selected, I still get paid.' Now, I meant that in a joking manner, but the point is that if I ask a player to do a repetition or I ask a player to do something, I'm asking them to do it for themselves and not for me. The players were able to understand then that, yes, I do care about them but, at the end of the day, they are doing everything for themselves and I am also doing everything I can to help them. Confidence in your own ability and your structured step-by-step return to play system is critical to this authority.

Understanding an athlete's internal motivators can also be a great way to keep them on track. An external motivator would be the natural reason why an athlete would do your rehab exercises. An external motivator might be so that he/she can get back to training and playing. But, the internal motivator is why that athlete plays in the first place and why it is important to him/her to get back playing. Having some understanding of these can help direct the athlete and keep the motivation present.

Another point worth mentioning is the relationship between the player and therapist. I would be very conscious of your relationship with players and coaches and avoid falling into the trap of thinking they are your friends. While this might sound brutally harsh, from my experience, when things start to go wrong for a player in professional sport, usually they will hang everybody else out to dry, even if it means using the therapist as a scapegoat. So just keep it in the back of your mind and never allow yourself to be caught off guard with a player/athlete. While athletes are great to work with, there is a thin line where you are a therapist and they are an athlete and that needs to be maintained at all times.

If you did have a scenario where a coach and/or athlete wants to go against your decision then ultimately you need to cover yourself with both the player and club. You need to document that you have explained the risks of playing and that, in your own expert opinion, you are against it. It is also worth notifying your superiors in the form of your CEO as ultimately that player is an asset to the club and it is your job to look after the healthcare of these assets. I would also notify my own coach that I will be letting the CEO know, purely to cover my own back and not in an attempt to undermine the coach. Being honest, logical and genuine with everything you do is of the utmost importance.

Luckily for me I've never had the experience (touch wood) of losing authority in my role at a club or with an athlete but I would strongly urge you that if you are in a situation where you are being undermined by players and coaches then it is time to have a look at how you carry yourself and how you speak to people, and to find ways of establishing authority back in those relationships. Establishing authority and maintaining authority in sport is absolutely vital yet very rarely spoken about. Unless you've got authority over players, unless you've got authority over the coach, then your injury prevention system will be very limited, from my experience. So now I hope you can see that we really need to have this whole package where it's not just one thing, but a series of interconnected things that are extremely important to the Injury Prevention Machine.

Summary of key points

How you speak and communicate to players and coaches is extremely important. You need to be able to communicate clearly and logically with confidence. Confidence comes from having clarity on the problem and the step-by-step treatment plan. Ensure you communicate on the coach's level so they understand how the consequences affect them and the team directly rather than focusing excessively on anatomical terms. Maintain your authority at all times while still being able to enjoy the company of your work colleagues.

CHAPTER 15

Putting it all together

So there you have it, the 12 micro systems that in my opinion need to be in place to give you the best shot possible of having a great injury prevention system and, ultimately, the best shot of having your athletes on the field/track.

To recap, we need every staff member to know their role and do their role extraordinarily.

The pre-season screening is screening for suitability to undergo the pre-season screening training loads and activities and not necessarily the sports-specific demands.

The pre-training markers need to be acted upon immediately in-play prior to the movement prep session.

The pre-training movement prep should essentially be a graded exposure to the loads that the athlete will face in the training after restoring an ability of all the major joints' tissues to lengthen and shorten as defined by the pre-training markers.

The on-feet loading needs to again follow a graded exposure with a common sense approach of reacting to the real world people in front of you without being afraid to deviate slightly if needs be. This will be particularly important for those athletes that return from injury and have some form of chronic load under their belts.

Moving well under load is a critical component in my opinion to a good injury prevention system. Weight must be distributed through the whole foot and hand and not just stuck on the heel of the foot or hand throughout the whole movement. An ability to challenge the base of support under load via the foot and hand is important to allow the nervous system to self-organise and react to perturbations accordingly. Move well in the gym, move well on the field.

Force absorption and in particular the ability to control one's body weight with efficient co-contractions at the knee and put the body in a good position to reapply force into the ground in various directions is still an area overlooked and not very well taught. A graded exposure deceleration programme from my experience will eliminate 'niggles' or 'flare-ups of old injuries', especially when training on 3G or different surfaces.

Soft tissue therapy can help desensitise perceived threats from the nervous system or can be just an excuse for an athlete to lie on the bed passively and look at their phone for half an hour. An ability to identify areas of perceived threat from the movement screens and pre-training markers gives direction to the soft tissue team and can make this time meaningful in attempting to restore homeostasis in the body while allowing the athlete to focus on their breathing and get back into rest and digest.

The acute injury management is also important to minimise the motor adaptations to pain or noxious stimulus. While the research is still emerging in this area, we want to ideally show the brain it is safe to load tissues in all directions within reason in a safe graded exposure manner. Asking why a non-contact injury has happened and why this tissue is overloading in the first place is a great place to start rectifying in the early days of an injury if we cannot do too much with the injured tissues. My own approach is to spend 80% of my time desensitising and gradually exposing the true stressor to load tolerance and to spend 20% of my time desensitising the symptomatic area with whatever means appropriate.

Pre-game movement prep should follow a logical graded exposure to the loads that the athlete will be expected to tolerate in the event themselves. This can be divided between movements performed in the changing room and on the field in conjunction with the strength and conditioning coach. All language used on game day is positive and designed to keep the athlete in the present moment.

The post-game approach is to overreact for the first 12 hours rather than under react and then begin to load to minimise motor adaptations to pain. While swelling is a natural process and required, the nervous system can react and produce excessive swelling which from my experience can be the reason for delayed progressions further down the line due to restricted range of motion, for example. We use compression aggressively post-game to minimise the overproduction of swelling and allow us to get the area moving and tolerating load safely in a graded manner as soon as possible.

Effective communication between all staff is important but especially between the medical and performance department. These practitioners need to be on the same page and saying the same things to the head coach. A conflicting message can lead to problems with on-feet loading amongst other things if the head coach is not clear on what needs to happen next. The communication should be at the level of the coach where they can see the consequences for their actions in their world rather than communicating in scientific terms.

Working towards doing these 12 components extraordinarily will give you a great shot of building momentum and each should complement the next to create a snowball effect.

If the athletes are moving well and are healthy, this allows the strength and conditioning coach to train the athlete hard but smart as well as building resilience and a chronic training load.

If the athlete is moving well in the gym with the strength and conditioning coach, this will help the medical department in dealing with reactions caused by excessive loads being absorbed in certain areas and pain or unpleasant sensations presenting in the treatment room.

If the therapist and strength and conditioning coaches work well together and communicate a common sense approach in logical terms to the head coach, then training loads can be managed smartly.

The medical and performance departments need to work well together to rehabilitate injured players to ensure they can tolerate appropriate loads when returning as well as having the confidence to produce force in as many directions as possible without any perceived threats or apprehension.

The components to an injury prevention programme are everyone's responsibility and not just those of one person or department. I hope you have found this resource useful in understanding my own injury prevention system that I have attempted to implement in professional sporting settings.

CHAPTER 16

Effective graded exposure when injuries do happen

While the 12 components above are important in my eyes in contributing towards preventing injuries, I believe there is another component that we have not talked about much in this book and that is adequate exposure to load when injuries or niggles do happen. If we appreciate the research in how the human body appears to react to pain or noxious stimulus, we should then be able to see the importance of giving the athlete back an ability to tolerate load through the injured limb in as many directions as possible.

While beyond the scope of this book and covered more in-depth in my other book, *The 'Go To' Physio*, I believe that if we adequately rehabilitate an athlete from previous injuries then we give ourselves a great chance of not seeing new injuries occur, ultimately as a result of altered loading strategies.

Therefore my approach is simple in that with every non-contact injury, we always start with the person's story and by asking what the nervous system perceives as a threat to the injured area at present.

There are usually three main stressors contributing to a pain experience:

1. **Physical stressors (Previous injuries)**
2. **Emotional stressors (Reactions in the diaphragm and pelvic floor)**
3. **Lifestyle stressors (Sleep, diet etc.)**

For me personally, a muscle tear or tendon injury is simply an overloading issue. The bigger question is WHY did this happen in the first place?

Why is that knee joint being overloaded in the first place?

Why is the nerve root becoming sensitised in the first place?

Why is that rotator cuff becoming painful and weak in the first place?

Why is the gluteus medius 'weak' in the first place?

The answer always lies in the person's story. If we can find the contributing stressors that we think are contributing to the pain experience or actual injury, desensitise these and expose them to load tolerances similar to the demands the athlete needs to tolerate, then we give ourselves a great chance of working smarter not harder by giving the athlete back movement variability and variance of movement.

The other important thing to mention at this point is we need to understand that the athlete may need to be exposed to higher loads before we see the movement strategies play out. Very often the basic musculoskeletal assessments of toe touching and single leg squats etc. may not expose the athletes tissues to enough load and speed of movement to expose the perceived threats still in the nervous system. Therefore, we truly need to expose our athletes to appropriate loads and speeds of movement that replicate the demands placed upon them in the real world.

Too often when therapists expose athletes to higher loads, they focus too much on the sagittal plane, for example, when there are still perceived threats present in the frontal and transverse planes.

The other big mistake when rehabilitating injuries is skipping steps. Too often I see athletes come to me after failing traditional approaches and going through the prolonged strength phases, yet still breaking down. It becomes clear when I take them through my graded exposure programme below that they have not earned the right to progress. For example before we worry about an athlete doing any hopping progressions, do they have the ability to co-contract at the knee joint and absorb load adequately through the whole limb? Or before that, can they manage a simple mini lunge and stick their body weight without excessive knee flexion and 'sinking'?

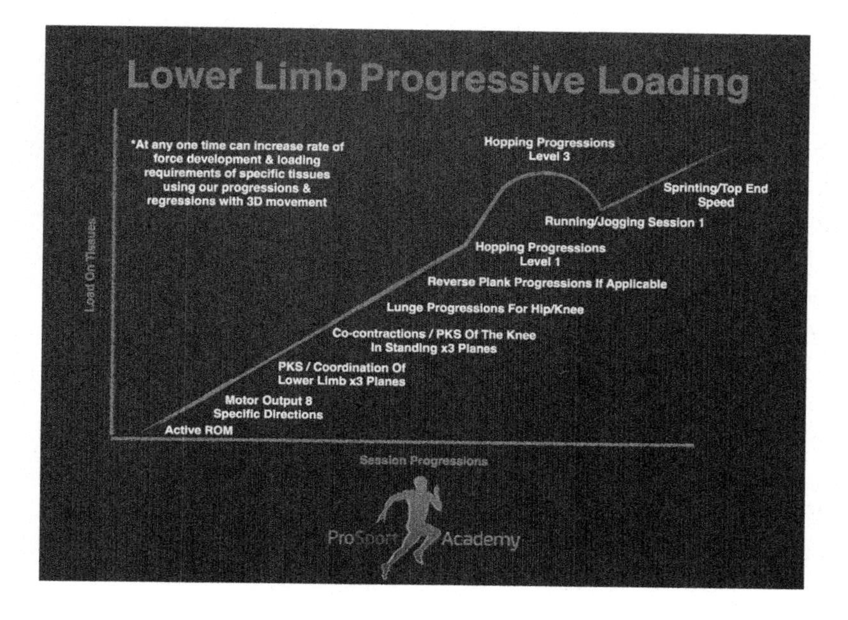

Here is an example of my lower limb progressive loading that I teach in my 'Go To' Therapist Mentorship. As you can see every single progression is the next logical progression. We build an ability to contract at the knee before even worrying about accepting body weight in standing. Once the athlete earns the right to progress, then we see minimal issues or setbacks. Although this loading programme looks generic, it is the information gained from the athlete's story combined with the assessment findings that is critical to giving us the directions that there are still perceived threats present.

Or worse, we go straight from single leg squats or lunges etc. straight to running progressions. This is a missed opportunity to build resilience to force absorption capabilities that will help when the athlete goes back into the team setting. Every progression should be the next logical progression and very often with even the most complex cases when we go back and decrease the perceived threat in the appropriate directions at each level, pain decreases, movement variability and variance of movement increases and the athlete's confidence begins to soar.

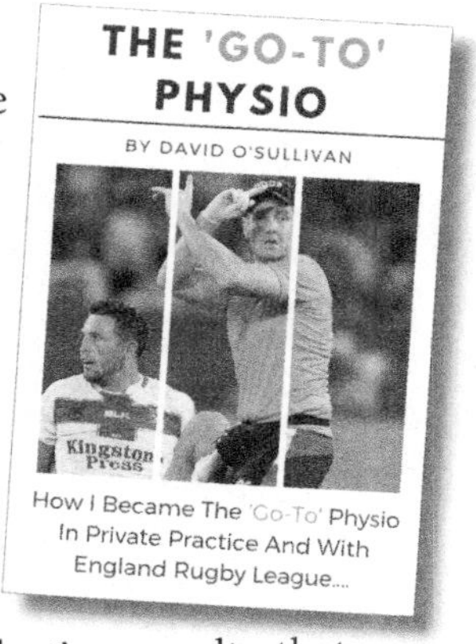

For a more in-depth view of my graded exposure system, please see my book, *The 'Go To' Physio Book.*

Your Opportunity To Work Personally With Dave

I would like to take a moment to say thank you for giving me your time and attention right up until the end of this book. It tells me you have the passion and desire to become the Go-To Therapist or Strength and Conditioning Coach in your area by first and foremost getting consistently great, long-lasting results that have a meaningful impact on your patients' or athletes' lives.

This is exactly the type of person that I love to work with, and because of that I am offering you an opportunity to continue to study with me personally.

1 Free Online Training

The Go-To Therapist Injury Prevention Case Study:

'How To Take A Group Of Athletes And Ensure They Are Resilient And Robust For The Demands Of Their Sport'

The Go-To Therapist Injury Prevention Case Study is a free and in-depth online training webinar that shows you step-by-step videos of how my system looks in the real world with patients and athletes. This 90-minute webinar will show you step by step (including example videos of exercises with real patients to look at) how people just like you have moved away from traditional physical therapy strategies of looking at the site of pain and strengthening it, which get some good results, to using the Go-To Therapist techniques that allow you to get consistent long-lasting results and then integrating these into movement prep sessions to ensure the results last.

You will see examples of everything you have just read in the pages of this book including the higher level deceleration progressions I use in both rehab settings and movement prep sessions. I will be hosting this free online training personally, and you will be able to submit your questions beforehand.

Here's what you will learn:

- **Step by step, the exact assessment, treatment and rehab system that Go-To Therapist students have used to add £12,000+ to their private practices within 90 days by increasing their retention, referrals, revenue and reputation by getting real world results with even the most tricky back pain cases.**
- **How to organise your movement screening for maximal efficiency without stress or being overwhelmed.**
- **How to interpret this information and implement it in the real world with movement prep progressions.**
- **How I progress my rehab and movement prep sessions in season to high level deceleration progressions.**
- **How to ensure your athletes are moving well in the gym.**

ACCESS THE FREE TRAINING HERE: **www.injurypreventionbook.com/webinar**

Choose this option if you want to see precisely how this system is being used by others just like you in pro sports and even by therapists working in private practice to increase retention, referrals and revenue. It is genuine training (90 minutes), and at the end of the training you will be given an opportunity to enrol in the Go-To Therapist Mentorship Programme, a 12-week Master Class where you can work personally with me if you decide it is right for you.

2 Work with me in the 12-week Go-To Therapist Online Mentorship Programme

The Go-To Therapist Mentorship Programme is a 12-week programme designed to help you build a Go-To Therapist practice in the quickest time possible, even if you are a new grad and have started up your own private practice, or to develop a treatment and step-by-step system in pro sport that looks at the person and not just the site of pain.

In my Go-To Therapist Mentorship I'll show you how to effortlessly get a patient highly motivated, and following every single progressive exercise you prescribe so you BOTH get the results you want using the exact same system I've used with thousands of professional athletes and my own private practice.

BUT you also get paid what you truly and ethically deserve and have the cannonball effect kick into your business of more RETENTION, REFERRALS, REVENUE and RECOGNITION with your REPUTATION as the Go-To Therapist cemented in your town or your sport.

How long are you going to continue treating patients knowing you could be giving a better service while also improving your caseload and massively growing your reputation and business?

This Online Go-To Therapist Mentorship Programme isn't about overtreating patients or bringing them for extra sessions when they don't need them but rather guiding them through a step-by-step progressive programme that allows them to build resilience for themselves while adding massive value to their lives.

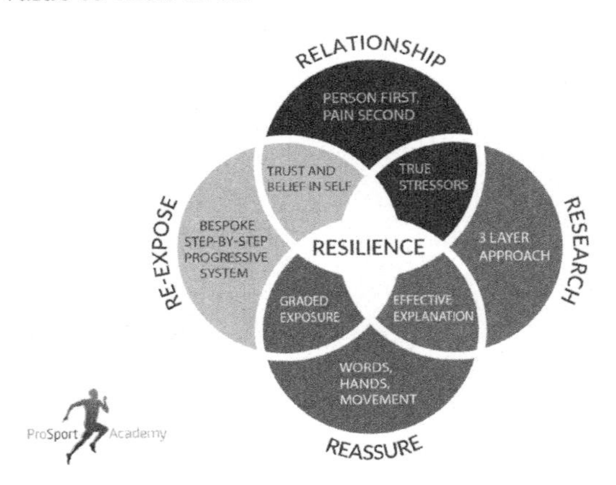

When you can get consistent, long-lasting results that add value to peoples' lives, you'll never have to worry about having a rollercoaster revenue each month, a quiet diary and patients cancelling or not showing up or your athletes breaking down when back in training.

The Go-To Therapist Mentorship Programme helps you gain a sound, clinically reasoned step-by-step process to treat the person in front of them looking at the body as a whole and bringing that person back to their ideal outcome successfully, be it returning to training or sport, or non-sporting patients returning to activities of daily living.

The online support and curriculum contains 12 modules (no longer than 1.5 hours per module) and the therapist has lifetime access to the content and support from me and my team. This contains my EXACT assessments, explanations, treatment techniques, rehab exercises, protocols and high-end rehab and performance exercises that I use on a daily basis with world-class athletes but also with my private practice patients.

The Therapist Mentorship will show you how to assess a patient using a simple common-sense approach, how to find the true stressors that are causing the symptomatic tissues/muscle/joint to overload and how to design a systematic step-by-step progressive treatment plan for that person's specific needs.

You will then learn how to EFFECTIVELY EXPLAIN your findings and the plan that needs to happen so that the patient can get the ideal result they want. This ensures the patient completely understands the plan and how they will progress during every session, which eliminates drop-offs and patients not adhering to exercises or feeling like they are not making progress.

From here you will learn how to use hands-on treatment techniques that are quick and effective and complement the rehab programme (so your patient does not get reliant on just soft tissue treatment) and how to progress the loading of the tissues (that are not doing enough) using a systematic approach that I have used successfully in pro sport for the past ten years.

By the fourth session (sometimes longer depending on the presentation) you will actually be exposing your patient to GREATER loads in a safe manner in the clinic by your movement choice.

They will need to be able to tolerate these in the real world with their first running session, for example. When they can do these movements without any nervous system motor adaptations, you will logically prove to yourself that your patient is READY to go back to running or lifting weights or picking up their kids, or whatever goal your patient has.

You will know your patient is READY to get back to doing what they love without setbacks, flare-ups or recurrence of injuries and you constantly second-guessing yourself.

Give me 1% of your time for 12 weeks and I'll help you achieve more than you achieved in the last three years

Everything you need is delivered to you via a series of instant access videos, PDF 'cheat sheets', live Q/A calls (with me), and an interactive online community (of hundreds of other Go-To Therapist students), all to ensure that you can put this system into your practice without any hassle or getting stuck.

ACCESS THE GO-TO THERAPIST MENTORSHIP HERE: www.thegotophysio.com/mentorship

If after reading this book you have decided that this type of method is exactly how you want to look at the body and get consistent real world results with your patients and athletes, and you do not want to wait another minute to have it working in your clinic or medical department, then go ahead and enroll in the programme now: **www.thegotophysio.com/mentorship**

The best part is that most of my students see a return on their investment in the programme before they even finish it. My aim is to add AT LEAST £12,000 to your annual revenue within 90 days through getting consistently great results and having super fans as your patients if you're in private practice or dramatically increasing your reputation and value in pro sport.

Are You A Strength & Conditioning Coach And Would Like Some Mentorship?

Or if you are a strength and conditioning coach and would like more in-depth mentoring on:

- Screening your athletes for gym programme planning
- Injury prevention techniques specific to strength coaches
- A sound step-by-step loading programme for injured athletes
- How to implement a step-by-step deceleration programme for health athletes without irritating old injuries
- And how to ensure your athletes are moving well in the gym with all the major lifts

then please visit

www.injurypreventionbook.com/strengthcoachmentor

So, what are you waiting for? Pick which one works best for you and let's get to work!

I'll see you on the webinar, in the advanced master class Go-To Therapist Mentorship Programme or brand new Strength and Conditioning Coach Mentorship.

To your professional success, your reputation and your patients' and athletes' improved quality of life and performance.

Dave O'Sullivan

Dave O'Sullivan

About Dave O'Sullivan

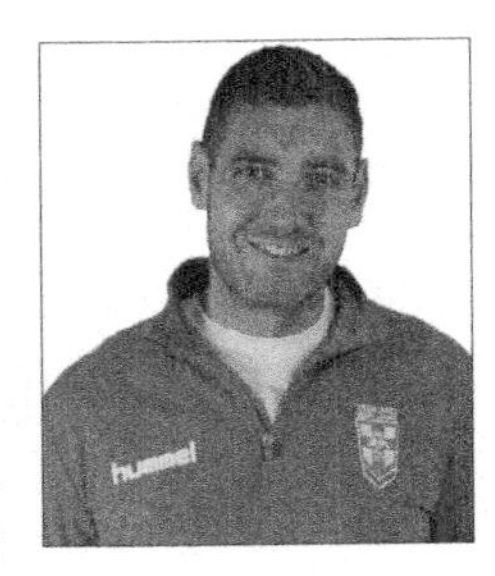

Dave O'Sullivan is a consultant rugby physiotherapist for England Rugby Union who has worked at the 2019 Rugby Union World Cup in Japan and the 2020 Six Nations. He was also the England Rugby League Physiotherapist for the 2017 Rugby League World Cup in Australia. Dave has the unique honor of being involved in a World Cup Final in Rugby League and Rugby Union.

Dave is the founder of The ProSport Academy Ltd. – an online mentoring company he set up to help therapists become the 'Go-To' Therapist in their area in 2015. Since 2015, Dave has worked with hundreds of professional sports physios, private practice therapists, strength coaches, rehab coaches and sports massage therapists with his method and systems helping people that have failed traditional approaches in clinics all over the world.

Dave also has grown ProSport Physiotherapy Huddersfield Ltd. – a successful private practice that helps both professional athletes and members of the general public get back to the things they love doing in life, pain-free from a one-room treatment room above a running shop to a five-treatment room private practice with a yoga studio and 10 full-time staff. Dave has now helped the therapists working in his clinic become the 'Go-To' Therapists in his own town of Huddersfield who make a meaningful impact on their patients' lives.

Dave is the host of the 'Go-To' Physio show (available on Youtube, Itunes, Soundcloud and Stitcher). The 'Go-To' Physio show helps therapists gain the confidence and clarity to get great, consistent long-lasting results that allow them to rapidly increase their retention, referrals, revenue and recognition as the 'Go-To' Therapist.

Dave is widely regarded as the 'Go-To' Therapist in Rugby League and consults with numerous clubs and athletes. He also works with professional golfers, GAA players and athletes in numerous other sports.

Every week, thousands of therapists receive his support/advice online and attend his seminars. His 'Go-To' Therapist Mentorship has sold out the past three times it has opened for enrollment.

REFERENCES

Key reference papers that have influenced my thought process

Blackburn, JT & Padua, DA. Influence of trunk flexion on hip and knee joint kinematics during a controlled drop landing. *Clin Biomech* (Bristol, Avon). 2008;23(3):313-9.

Bosch, F & Van Hooren, B. Influence of Muscle Slack on High-Intensity Sport Performance: A Review. *Strength And Conditioning Journal.* 2016;38(5),75-87.

Chaudhry, H, Schleip, R, Ji Z, Bukiet B, Maney M, Findley T. Three-dimensional mathematical model for deformation of human fasciae in manual therapy. *J Am Osteopath Assoc.* 2008;108(8):379-90.

Courtney, R. The functions of breathing and its dysfunctions and their relationship to breathing therapy. *International Journal of Osteopathic Medicine.* 2009;12(3),78-85.

Dyhre-Poulsen P, Krogsgaard MR. Muscular reflexes elicited by electrical stimulation of the anterior cruciate ligament in humans. *J Appl Physiol.* 2000;89(6):2191-5.

Farina D, Arendt-Nielsen L, Graven-Nielsen T. Experimental muscle pain reduces initial motor unit discharge rates during sustained submaximal contractions. *J Appl Physiol.* 2005;98(3):999-1005.

Fukui T, Otake Y, Kondo T. In which direction does skin move during joint movement? *Skin Res Technol.* 2016;22(2):181-8.

Gregory JE, Wise AK, Wood SA, Prochazka A, Proske U. Muscle history, fusimotor activity and the human stretch reflex. *J Physiol* (Lond). 1998;513(Pt 3):927-34.

Harper CJ, Shahgholi L, Cieslak K, Hellyer NJ, Strommen JA, Boon AJ. Variability in diaphragm motion during normal breathing, assessed with B-mode ultrasound. *J Orthop Sports Phys Ther.* 2013;43(12):927-31.

Hodges PW, Coppieters MW, Macdonald D, Cholewicki J. New insight into motor adaptation to pain revealed by a combination of modelling and empirical approaches. *Eur J Pain.* 2013;17(8):1138-46.

Hodges PW, Ervilha UF, Graven-Nielsen T. Changes in motor unit firing rate in synergist muscles cannot explain the maintenance of force during constant force painful contractions. *J Pain.* 2008;9(12):1169-74.

Hodges PW, Smeets RJ. Interaction between pain, movement, and physical activity: short-term benefits, long-term consequences, and targets for treatment. *Clin J Pain.* 2015;31(2):97-107.

Hug F, Hodges PW, Carroll TJ, De martino E, Magnard J, Tucker K. Motor Adaptations to Pain during a Bilateral Plantarflexion Task: Does the Cost of Using the Non-Painful Limb Matter? *PLOS ONE.* 2016;11(4):e0154524.

Hug F, Hodges PW, Tucker K. Task dependency of motor adaptations to an acute noxious stimulation. *J Neurophysiol.* 2014;111(11):2298-306.

Johansson H, Sjölander P, Sojka P. Receptors in the knee joint ligaments and their role in the biomechanics of the joint. *Crit Rev Biomed Eng.* 1991;18(5):341-68.

Maas H, Baan GC, Huijing PA. Muscle force is determined also by muscle relative position: isolated effects. *J Biomech.* 2004;37(1):99-110.

Mason-Mackay AR, Whatman C, Reid D. The effect of reduced ankle dorsiflexion on lower extremity mechanics during landing: A systematic review. *J Sci Med Sport.* 2017;20(5):451-458.

Morin JB, Gimenez P, Edouard P, et al. Sprint Acceleration Mechanics: The Major Role of Hamstrings in Horizontal Force Production. *Front Physiol.* 2015;6:404.

Moritz CT, Farley CT. Passive dynamics change leg mechanics for an unexpected surface during human hopping. *J Appl Physiol.* 2004;97(4):1313-22.

Moseley GL, Hodges PW. Reduced variability of postural strategy prevents normalization of motor changes induced by back pain: a risk factor for chronic trouble? *Behav Neurosci.* 2006;120(2):474-6.

Prior S, Mitchell T, Whiteley R, et al. The influence of changes in trunk and pelvic posture during single leg standing on hip and thigh muscle activation in a pain free population. *BMC Sports Sci Med Rehabil.* 2014;6(1):13.

Roeder BA, Kokini K, Sturgis JE, Robinson JP, Voytik-Harbin SL. Tensile mechanical properties of three-dimensional type I collagen extracellular matrices with varied microstructure. *J Biomech Eng.* 2002;124(2):214-22.

Scarfe AC, Li FX, Reddin DB, Bridge MW. A new progression scale for common lower-limb rehabilitation tasks. *J Strength Cond Res.* 2011;25(3):612-9.

Schleip R, Naylor IL, Ursu D, et al. Passive muscle stiffness may be influenced by active contractility of intramuscular connective tissue. *Med Hypotheses.* 2006;66(1):66-71.

Shacklock MO. Central pain mechanisms: A new horizon in manual therapy. *Aust J Physiother.* 1999;45(2):83-92.

Sokoloff AJ, Siegel SG, Cope TC. Recruitment order among motoneurons from different motor nuclei. *J Neurophysiol.* 1999;81(5):2485-92.

Solomonow M. Ligaments: a source of work-related musculoskeletal disorders. *J Electromyogr Kinesiol.* 2004;14(1):49-60.

Tanaka H, Ikezoe T, Umehara J, et al. Influences of Fascicle Length During Isometric Training on Improvement of Muscle Strength. *J Strength Cond Res.* 2016;30(11):3249-3255.

Teng HL, Powers CM. Hip-Extensor Strength, Trunk Posture, and Use of the Knee-Extensor Muscles During Running. *J Athl Train.* 2016;51(7):519-24.

Teng HL, Powers CM. Influence of trunk posture on lower extremity energetics during running. *Med Sci Sports Exerc.* 2015;47(3):625-30.

Teyhen DS, Shaffer SW, Butler RJ, et al. What Risk Factors Are Associated With Musculoskeletal Injury in US Army Rangers? A Prospective Prognostic Study. *Clin Orthop Relat Res.* 2015;473(9):2948-58.

Thacker, M. Louis Gifford – Revolutionary: The Mature Organism Model, an embodied cognitive perspective of pain. *In Touch.* 2015;152 (1), p4-9.

Tucker KJ, Hodges PW. Changes in motor unit recruitment strategy during pain alters force direction. *Eur J Pain.* 2010;14(9):932-8.

Tucker K, Hodges PW, Van den hoorn W, Nordez A, Hug F. Does stress within a muscle change in response to an acute noxious stimulus? *PLOS ONE.* 2014;9(3):e91899.

Van der krogt MM, De graaf WW, Farley CT, Moritz CT, Richard casius LJ, Bobbert MF. Robust passive dynamics of the musculoskeletal system compensate for unexpected surface changes during human hopping. *J Appl Physiol.* 2009;107(3):801-8.

Verkuil B, Brosschot JF, Tollenaar MS, Lane RD, Thayer JF. Prolonged Non-metabolic Heart Rate Variability Reduction as a Physiological Marker of Psychological Stress in Daily Life. *Ann Behav Med.* 2016;50(5):704-714.

Printed in Great Britain
by Amazon